Land Mark Clinical Trials in Cardiology

Mossaab Shuraih, MD. CCDS.
Clinical Cardiac Electrophysiology
Texas Heart Institute / Texas Heart Rhtyhm Center
Houston, Texas.

Zaher Fanari, MD.
Cardiology fellow
Christiana Care Health System
Newark, Delaware.

.

All rights reserved
Mossaab Shuraih MD.
Land Mark Clinical Trials in Cardiology.
ISBN: 978-0-9899496-0-6

© 2013, M. Shuraih.
Publication of Mo Medical Consulting LLC.
Momedicalco@gmail.com

Preface

During my CCU rounds as a first year cardiology fellow, my attending asked me: what was the trial that showed Aspirin to be beneficial in the acute myocardial infarction? I have read something about that trial a while back, but the only thing I could recall at that moment was that the trial acronym had the number "2" and two letters "i" in it so TIMI-2 seemed to be a reasonable answer to me at that moment, and of course I was wrong!

First I did a small sketch to help me memorize that trial, and the idea of this book was born. I wanted to have a quick reference in an-easy-to-remember manner containing the most needed-to-know trials for students starting to learn about the evidence-based practice in the cardiovascular disease. Soon thereafter, I realized that if I want to demonstrate all the trials that fell between my hands, I have to sketch over 500 trials, besides time restrictions, I believed including large number of trials will defeat the purpose of consolidating the most relevant trials in one piece of work.

With a lot of help from my colleagues and attendings, we chose the trials that are presented in this book, little over 130 clinical trials. Having done so, I may have inadvertently omitted important trials or included a less relevant one with more catchy acronym. However, speaking as a student of the field, not only as an author, this book was a good start and a helpful tool that worked as a foundation upon which I was able to build and expand my understanding and knowledge in cardiovascular medicine, and I hope it will provide the same benefits to other medical professionals as well.

Mossaab Shuraih MD. CCDS.

Acknowledgement

This work was inspired by Dr. Craig M. Pratt.
Most of the abstract summaries and organizations were done by Dr Zaher Fanari.
Sketches of ESCAPE, RALES, and 4S trials were done by Dr Christian Assad.

Contributors

Christian Assad, MD
Zaher Fanari, MD
Syed Gilani, MD
Mazen Hadid, MD
Jennifer M. Lopez, MD
Miguel Valderrabano, MD

About this book

This book serves as a quick reference and memory-aid tool for the acronyms and the major findings of some of the major trials in the cardiovascular field. The trial acronym is demonstrated with a cartoon sketch that represents the trial; or merely demonstrates the acronym and tries to link it, in a visual manner, to the trial.

The trial abstracts with the appropriate references are provided as well. This book is a good starting point for medical trainees to become familiar with evidence-based medicine of the cardiovascular disease. However, complete review and understanding of the full texts of the trials, not merely the abstracts, is a must. In acdition, the fast pace at which the field is growing, major trials is being conducted every year, with constant changes and updates to the guidelines, and one must keep in mind such limitations when looking at this work.

Disclaimer

This book is to be used for educational purposes, The book functions as a quick reference to some of the most relevant clinical trials in cardiology. Other relevant clinical trials may not be demonstrated in this book. This book does not represent the current guidelines in the cardiovascular field. For the most current recommendations and guidelines please refer to the appropriate sources. No medical recommendations or management decisions should be based on the content of this book. We apologize for any inadvertent mistakes or misinterpretations that might be found, we will be happy to correct them in future reprints.

Abbreviation:

AAD   Antiarrhythmic drug
ACEI   Angiotensin-converting-enzyme inhibitor
ACS   Acute coronary syndrome
AF   Atrial fibrillation
ARB   Angiotensin receptor antagonist
BB   Beta blockers
BiV   Biventricular pacing
BNP   Brain natriuretic peptide
CABG   Coronary artery bypass graft
CAD   Coronary artery disease
CCB   Calcium channel blocker
CHF   Congestive heart failure
CVD   Cardiovascular disease
DES   Drug-eluting stent
DM   Diabetes mellitus
ED   Emergency department
EF   Ejection fraction
EP   Electrophysiology
ER   Emergency room
GP   Glycoproteins
HCTZ   Hydrochlorothiazide
HF   Heart failure
HLP   Hyperlipidemia
HTN   Hypertension
ICD   Implantable cardioverter-defibrillator
LA   Left atrium
LV   Left ventricle
LVEF   Left ventricular ejection fraction
MI   Myocardial infarct
NSTEMI   Non-ST elevation myocardial infarction
NYHA   New york heart association
OPT   Optimal pharmacologic therapy
PCI   Percutaneous coronary intervention
PPM   Permanent pacemaker
RA   Right atrium
RV   Right ventricle
STEMI   ST elevation myocardial infarction
TAVI   Transcatheter aortic-valve implantation
UA   Unstable angina
UFH   Unfractionated heparin
VT   Ventricular tachycardia

CHAPTERS   **Page**

Table of contents :

Electrophysiology Trials

Miscellaneous Trials

ST-Elevation Myocardial Infarction (STEMI) Trials.

ISIS-2 TRIAL

RANDOMISED TRIAL OF INTRAVENOUS STREPTOKINASE, ORAL ASPIRIN, BOTH, OR NEITHER AMONG 17,187 CASES OF SUSPECTED ACUTE MYOCARDIAL INFARCTION: ISIS-2.
LANCET. 1988.

This trial was done at the early days of coronary reperfusion using Streptokinase (1988). In ISIS-II patients with suspected acute MI were randomized to receive either Aspirin alone for a month, Streptokinase alone, both aspirin and streptokinase, or neither treatment. The interesting finding was that Aspirin alone was as good as streptokinase alone in reducing vascular mortality at 5 weeks. The combination of streptokinase and aspirin was significantly better than either agent alone, and this early survival advantages, was also maintained in a 10-year follow up study published in 1998.

RamISIS-II had two faithful servants little Apirino and Sterptokina

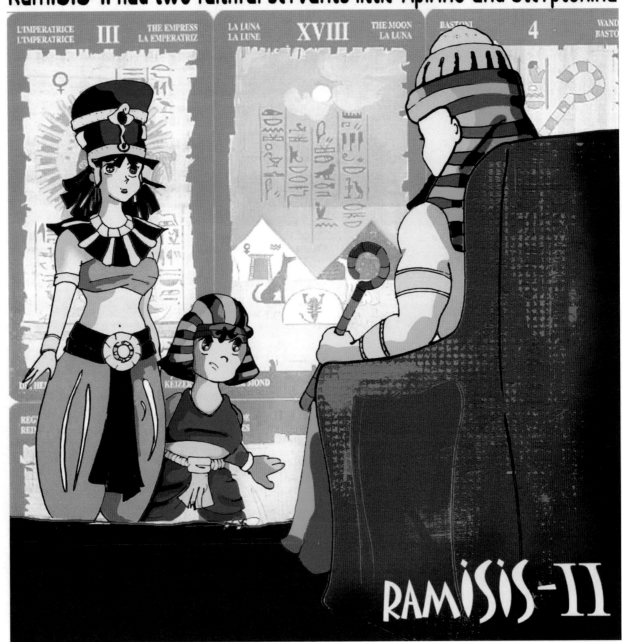

ISIS-2 TRIAL

Randomised trial of intravenous streptokinase, oral aspirin, both, or neither among 17,187 cases of suspected acute myocardial infarction: ISIS-2. ISIS-2 (Second International Study of Infarct Survival) Collaborative Group

Lancet. 1988; August 13; 2(8607):349-60.

17,187 patients entering 417 hospitals up to 24 hours (median 5 hours) after the onset of suspected acute myocardial infarction were randomised, with placebo control, between: (i) a 1-hour intravenous infusion of 1.5 MU of streptokinase; (ii) one month of 160 mg/day enteric-coated aspirin; (iii) both active treatments; or (iv) neither. Streptokinase alone and aspirin alone each produced a highly significant reduction in 5-week vascular mortality: 791/8592 (9.2%) among patients allocated streptokinase infusion vs 1029/8595 (12.0%) among those allocated placebo infusion (odds reduction: 25% SD 4; 2p less than 0.00001); 804/8587 (9.4%) vascular deaths among patients allocated aspirin tablets vs 1016/8600 (11.8%) among those allocated placebo tablets (odds reduction: 23% SD 4; 2p less than 0.00001). The combination of streptokinase and aspirin was significantly (2p less than 0.0001) better than either agent alone. Their separate effects on vascular deaths appeared to be additive: 343/4292 (8.0%) among patients allocated both active agents vs 568/4300 (13.2%) among those allocated neither (odds reduction: 42% SD 5; 95% confidence limits 34-50%). There was evidence of benefit from each agent even for patients treated late after pain onset (odds reductions at 0-4, 5-12, and 13-24 hours: 35% SD 6, 16% SD 7, and 21% SD 12 for streptokinase alone; 25% SD 7, 21% SD 7, and 21% SD 12 for aspirin alone; and 53% SD 8, 32% SD 9, and 38% SD 15 for the combination of streptokinase and aspirin). Streptokinase was associated with an excess of bleeds requiring transfusion (0.5% vs 0.2%) and of confirmed cerebral haemorrhage (0.1% vs 0.0%), but with fewer other strokes (0.6% vs 0.8%). These "other" strokes may have included a few undiagnosed cerebral haemorrhages, but still there was no increase in total strokes (0.7% streptokinase vs 0.8% placebo infusion). Aspirin significantly reduced non-fatal reinfarction (1.0% vs 2.0%) and non-fatal stroke (0.3% vs 0.6%), and was not associated with any significant increase in cerebral haemorrhage or in bleeds requiring transfusion. An excess of non-fatal reinfarction was reported when streptokinase was used alone, but this appeared to be entirely avoided by the addition of aspirin. Those allocated the combination of streptokinase and aspirin had significantly fewer reinfarctions (1.8% vs 2.9%), strokes (0.6% vs 1.1%), and deaths (8.0% vs 13.2%) than those allocated neither. The differences in vascular and in all-cause mortality produced by streptokinase and by aspirin remain highly significant (2p less than 0.001 for each) after the median of 15 months of follow-up thus far available.

ISIS-2: 10 year survival among patients with suspected acute myocardial infarction in randomised comparison of intravenous streptokinase, oral aspirin, both, or neither. The ISIS-2 (Second International Study of Infarct Survival) Collaborative Group. Baigent C et al.

British Medical Association (BMJ). 1998; May 2; 316(7141):1337-43.

OBJECTIVE
To assess effects of intravenous streptokinase, one month of oral aspirin, or both, on long term survival after suspected acute myocardial infarction.

DESIGN: Randomised, "2 x 2 factorial," placebo controlled trial.

SETTING: 417 hospitals in 16 countries.

SUBJECTS: 17 187 patients with suspected acute myocardial infarction randomised between March 1985 and December 1987. Follow up of vital status complete to at least 1 January 1990 for 95% of all patients and to mid-1997 for the 6213 patients in United Kingdom.

INTERVENTIONS: Intravenous streptokinase (1.5 MU in 1 hour) and oral aspirin (162 mg daily for 1 month) versus matching placebos.

MAIN OUTCOME MEASURES: Mortality from all causes during up to 10 years' follow up, with subgroup analyses based on 4 year follow up.

RESULTS: After randomisation, 1841 deaths were recorded in days 0-35, 991 from day 36 to end of year 1, 1478 in years 2-4, and 1230 in years 5-10. Allocation to streptokinase was associated with 29 (95% confidence interval 20 to 38) fewer deaths per 1000 patients during days 0-35. This early benefit persisted (death rate ratio 0.98 (0.92 to 1.04) for additional deaths between day 36 and end of year 10), so that there were 28 (14 to 42) and 23 (2 to 44) fewer deaths per 1000 patients treated with streptokinase after 4 years and 10 years respectively. There was no evidence that absolute survival benefit increased with prolonged follow up among any category of patient, including those presenting early after symptoms started or with anterior ST elevation. Nor did the early benefits seem to be lost in any category (including those aged over 70). Allocation to one month of aspirin was associated with 26 (16 to 35) fewer deaths per 1000 during first 35 days, with little further benefit or loss during subsequent years (death rate ratio 0.99 (0.93 to 1.06) between day 36 and end of year 10). The early benefit obtained with combination of streptokinase and one month of aspirin also seemed to persist long term.

CONCLUSIONS: The early survival advantages produced by fibrinolytic therapy and one month of aspirin started in acute myocardial infarction seem to be maintained for at least 10 years.

CARS AND CHAMP TRIALS

Both CHAMP and CARS trials showed that low dose warfarin, combined with 81 mg of aspirin, does not provide any additional benefit, in patients post acute myocardial infarction, over aspirin 160 mg daily alone.

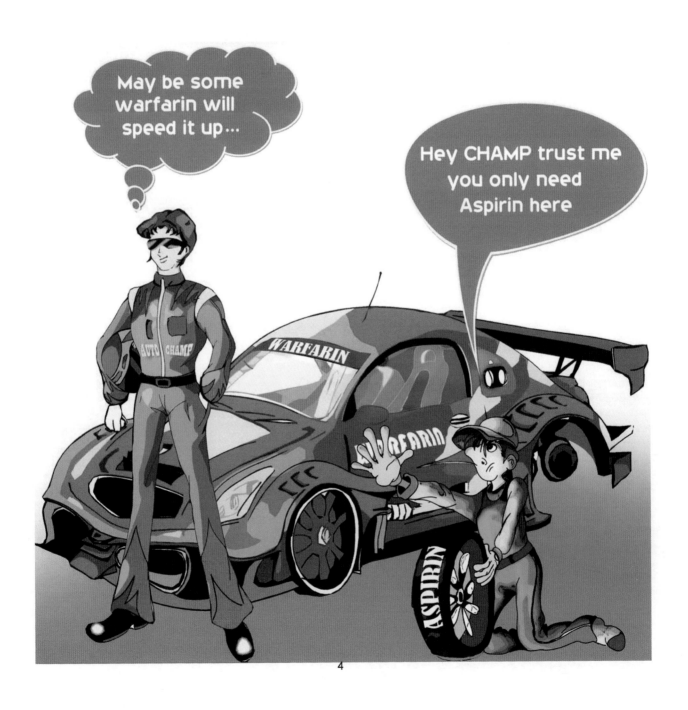

CARS TRIAL

Randomised double-blind trial of fixed low-dose warfarin with aspirin after myocardial infarction. Coumadin Aspirin Reinfarction Study (CARS) Investigators.

Lancet. 1997. August; 9; 350(9075):389-96.

BACKGROUND

Antiplatelet therapy with aspirin and systematic anticoagulation with warfarin reduce cardiovascular morbidity and mortality after myocardial infarction when given alone. In the Coumadin Aspirin Reinfarction Study (CARS), we aimed to find out whether a combination of low-dose warfarin and low-dose aspirin would give superior results to standard aspirin monotherapy without excessive bleeding risk.

METHODS

We used a randomised double-blind study design. At 293 sites, we randomly assigned 8803 patients who had had myocardial infarction, treatment with 160 mg aspirin, 3 mg warfarin with 80 mg aspirin, or 1 mg warfarin with 80 mg aspirin. Patients took a single tablet daily, and attended for prothrombin time (PT) measurements at weeks 1, 2, 3, 4, 6, and 12, and then every 3 months. Patients were followed up for a maximum of 33 months (median 14 months).

FINDINGS

The primary event was first occurrence of reinfarction, non-fatal ischaemic stroke, or cardiovascular death. 1-year life-table estimates for the primary event were 8.6% (95% CI 7.6-9.6) for 160 mg aspirin, 8.4% (7.4-9.4) for 3 mg warfarin with 80 mg aspirin, and 8.8% (7.6-10) for 1 mg warfarin with 80 mg aspirin. Primary comparisons were done with all follow-up data. The relative risk of the primary event for the 160 mg aspirin group compared with the 3 mg warfarin with 80 mg aspirin group was 0.95 (0.81-1.12, p = 0.57). For spontaneous major haemorrhage (not procedure related), 1-year life-table estimates were 0.74% (0.43-1.1) in the 160 mg aspirin group and 1.4% (0.94-1.8) in the 3 mg warfarin with 80 mg aspirin group (p = 0.014 log rank on follow-up). For the 3382 patients assigned 3 mg warfarin with 80 mg aspirin, the INR results were: at week 1 (n = 2985) median 1.51 (IQR 1.23-2.13); at week 4 (n = 2701) 1.27 (1.13-1.64); at month 6 (n = 2145) 1.19 (1.08-1.44).

INTERPRETATION

Low, fixed-dose warfarin (1 mg or 3 mg) combined with low-dose aspirin (80 mg) in patients who have had myocardial infarction does not provide clinical benefit beyond that achievable with 160 mg aspirin monotherapy.

CHAMP TRIAL

Department of Veterans Affairs Cooperative Studies Program Clinical Trial comparing combined warfarin and aspirin with aspirin alone in survivors of acute myocardial infarction: primary results of the CHAMP study.

Fiore LD, et al.

Circulation. 2002. February;5;105(5):557-63.

BACKGROUND

Both aspirin and warfarin when used alone are effective in the secondary prevention of vascular events and death after acute myocardial infarction. We tested the hypothesis that aspirin and warfarin therapy, when combined, would be more effective than aspirin monotherapy.

Methods and Results

We conducted a randomized open-label study to compare the efficacy of warfarin (target international normalized ratio 1.5 to 2.5 IU) plus aspirin (81 mg daily) with the efficacy of aspirin monotherapy (162 mg daily) in reducing the total mortality in 5059 patients enrolled within 14 days of infarction and followed for a median of 2.7 years. Secondary end points included recurrent myocardial infarction, stroke, and major hemorrhage. Four hundred thirty-eight (17.3%) of 2537 patients assigned to the aspirin group and 444 (17.6%) of 2522 patients assigned to the combination group died (log-rank P=0.76). Recurrent myocardial infarction occurred in 333 patients (13.1%) taking aspirin and in 336 patients (13.3%) taking combination therapy (log-rank P=0.78). Stroke occurred in 89 patients (3.5%) taking aspirin and in 79 patients (3.1%) taking combination therapy (log-rank P=0.52). Major bleeding occurred more frequently in the combination therapy group than in the aspirin group (1.28 versus 0.72 events per 100 person years of follow-up, respectively; P<0.001). There were 14 individuals with intracranial bleeds in both the aspirin and combination therapy groups.

CONCLUSIONS

In post-myocardial infarction patients, warfarin therapy (at a mean international normalized ratio of 1.8) combined with low-dose aspirin did not provide a clinical benefit beyond that achievable with aspirin monotherapy.

AIR-PAMI TRIAL

A RANDOMIZED TRIAL OF TRANSFER FOR PRIMARY ANGIOPLASTY VERSUS ON-SITE THROMBOLYSIS IN PATIENTS WITH HIGH-RISK MYOCARDIAL INFARCTION: THE AIR PRIMARY ANGIOPLASTY IN MYOCARDIAL INFARCTION STUDY. GRINES CL, ET AL.

Journal of the American College of Cardiology(JACC). 2002; June 5; 39(11):1713-9

This trial was done to see whether transferring a patient with AMI to a center capable of PCI will offer any benefit over using fibrinolytic at a site that does not have that ability. Patients were randomized to either stay at the center and get fibrinolytic agent or transfer to a PCI center. AIR-PAMI trial showed that patients with high-risk AMI at hospitals without a catheterization laboratory may have an improved outcome when transferred for primary PTCA versus on-site thrombolysis; however because of the inability to recruit the necessary sample size, this did not achieve statistical significance.

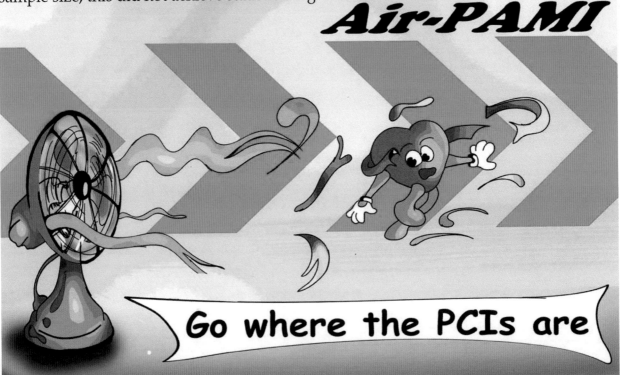

Air-PAMI

Go where the PCIs are

OBJECTIVES: The Air Primary Angioplasty in Myocardial Infarction (PAMI) study was designed to determine the best reperfusion strategy for patients with high-risk acute myocardial infarction (AMI) at hospitals without percutaneous transluminal coronary angioplasty (PTCA) capability.

BACKGROUND: Previous studies have suggested that high-risk patients have better outcomes with primary PTCA than with thrombolytic therapy. It is unknown whether this advantage would be lost if the patient had to be transferred for PTCA, and reperfusion was delayed.

METHODS: Patients with high-risk AMI (age >70 years, anterior MI, Killip class II/III, heart rate >100 beats/min or systolic BP <100 mm Hg) who were eligible for thrombolytic therapy were randomized to either transfer for primary PTCA or on-site thrombolysis.

RESULTS: One hundred thirty-eight patients were randomized before the study ended (71 to transfer for PTCA and 67 to thrombolysis). The time from arrival to treatment was delayed in the transfer group (155 vs. 51 min, p < 0.0001), largely due to the initiation of transfer (43 min) and transport time (26 min). Patients randomized to transfer had a reduced hospital stay (6.1 +/- 4.3 vs. 7.5 +/- 4.3 days, p = 0.015) and less ischemia (12.7% vs. 31.8%, p = 0.007). At 30 days, a 38% reduction in major adverse cardiac events was observed for the transfer group; however, because of the inability to recruit the necessary sample size, this did not achieve statistical significance (8.4% vs. 13.6%, p = 0.331).

CONCLUSIONS: Patients with high-risk AMI at hospitals without a catheterization laboratory may have an improved outcome when transferred for primary PTCA versus on-site thrombolysis; however, this will require further study. The marked delay in the transfer process suggests a role for triaging patients directly to specialized heart-attack centers.

PRAGUE TRIAL AND DANISH TRIAL IN ACUTE MYOCARDIAL INFARCTION-2 (DANAMI-2)

PRAGUE and DANAMI-2 were European trials, and they were among the first trials to demonstrated that transporting patients to an angioplasty capable center in the acute phase of myocardial infarction is safe and feasible strategy. And it showed that, if the transportation was done within 2 hours of the presentation, it is superior in clinical outcomes to on-site fibrinolysis.

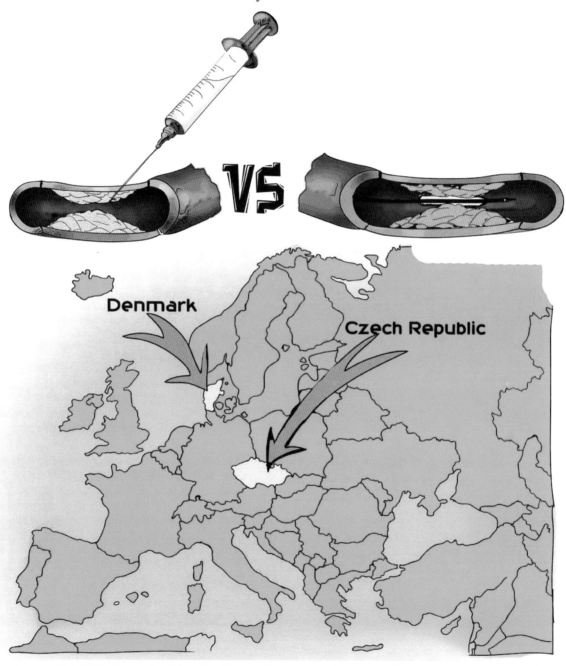

Both DANAMI-2 and PRAGUE trials were done in Europe to compared PCI versus thrombolytic. DANAMI was done in Denmark and PRAGUE is the capital of the Czech Republic where PRAGUE trial was performed.

PRAGUE TRIAL

Multicentre randomized trial comparing transport to primary angioplasty vs immediate thrombolysis vs combined strategy for patients with acute myocardial infarction presenting to a community hospital without a catheterization laboratory. The PRAGUE study. Widimsk P et al.

European heart journal 2000; May 21; (10):823-31.

BACKGROUND

Primary coronary angioplasty is an effective reperfusion strategy in acute myocardial infarction. However, its availability is limited, and transporting patients to an angioplasty centre in the acute phase of myocardial infarction has not yet been proved safe.

METHODS

The PRAGUE study (PRimary Angioplasty in patients transferred from General community hospitals to specialized PTCA Units with or without Emergency thrombolysis) compared three reperfusion strategies in patients with acute myocardial infarction, presenting within 6 h of symptom onset at community hospitals without a catheterization laboratory: group A - thrombolytic therapy in community hospitals (n=99), group B -thrombolytic therapy during transportation to angioplasty (n=100), group C - immediate transportation for primary angioplasty without pre-treatment with thrombolysis (n=101).

RESULTS

No complications occurred during transportation in group C. Two ventricular fibrillations occurred during transportation in group B. Median admission-reperfusion time in transported patients (group B 106 min, group C 96 min) compared favourably with the anticipated >90 min in group A. The combined primary end-point (death/reinfarction/stroke at 30 days) was less frequent in group C (8%) compared to groups B (15%) and A (23%, P<0. 02). The incidence of reinfarction was markedly reduced by transport to primary angioplasty (1% in group C vs 7% in group B vs 10% in group A, P<0.03).

CONCLUSIONS

Transferring patients from community hospitals to a tertiary angioplasty centre in the acute phase of myocardial infarction is feasible and safe. This strategy is associated with a significant reduction in the incidence of reinfarction and the combined clinical end-point of death/reinfarction/stroke at 30 days when compared to standard thrombolytic therapy at the community hospital.

DANish trial in Acute Myocardial Infarction-2 (DANAMI-2).Trial

A comparison of coronary angioplasty with fibrinolytic therapy in acute myocardial infarction. Andersen HR et al

New England Journal of Medicine (NEJM) 2003; August 21; 349:733-42

BACKGROUND

For the treatment of myocardial infarction with ST-segment elevation, primary angioplasty is considered superior to fibrinolysis for patients who are admitted to hospitals with angioplasty facilities. Whether this benefit is maintained for patients who require transportation from a community hospital to a center where invasive treatment is available is uncertain.

METHODS

We randomly assigned 1572 patients with acute myocardial infarction to treatment with angioplasty or accelerated treatment with intravenous alteplase; 1129 patients were enrolled at 24 referral hospitals and 443 patients at 5 invasive-treatment centers. The primary study end point was a composite of death, clinical evidence of reinfarction, or disabling stroke at 30 days.

RESULTS

Among patients who underwent randomization at referral hospitals, the primary end point was reached in 8.5 percent of the patients in the angioplasty group, as compared with 14.2 percent of those in the fibrinolysis group (P=0.002). The results were similar among patients who were enrolled at invasive-treatment centers: 6.7 percent of the patients in the angioplasty group reached the primary end point, as compared with 12.3 percent in the fibrinolysis group (P=0.05). Among all patients, the better outcome after angioplasty was driven primarily by a reduction in the rate of reinfarction (1.6 percent in the angioplasty group vs. 6.3 percent in the fibrinolysis group, P<0.001); no significant differences were observed in the rate of death (6.6 percent vs. 7.8 percent, P=0.35) or the rate of stroke (1.1 percent vs. 2.0 percent, P=0.15). Ninety-six percent of patients were transferred from referral hospitals to an invasive-treatment center within two hours.

CONCLUSIONS

A strategy for reperfusion involving the transfer of patients to an invasive-treatment center for primary angioplasty is superior to on-site fibrinolysis, provided that the transfer takes two hours or less.

COMMIT/CCS-2

CLOPIDOGREL AND METOPROLOL IN MYOCARDIAL INFARCTION TRIAL) COLLABORATIVE GROUP
Lancet. 2005.

The Clopidogrel and Metoprolol in Myocardial Infarction Trial/Second Chinese Cardiac Study (COMMIT/CCS-2) is the largest clinical study ever conducted in China. The study enrolled 45,852 patients with suspected acute MI, and it had two arms one to evaluate the effect of clopidogrel, while the other arm studied the effect of IV metoprolol in patients with acute MI.

The Clopidogrel arm was one of the first studies to show the benefit of adding Clopidogrel to aspirin in patients presented with acute MI. Patients were randomized to receive clopidogrel 75 mg once daily or placebo. The study showed significant reduction in mortality with clopidogrel treatment without any increase in bleeding. While in the metoprolol arm, patients were randomized within 24 hours of symptom onset to receive metoprolol IV followed by the oral beta blocker. It turned out that the IV beta blocker reduces the risk of in-hospital reinfarction, but on the expense of increased risk of cardiogenic shock, with no overall survival benefit.

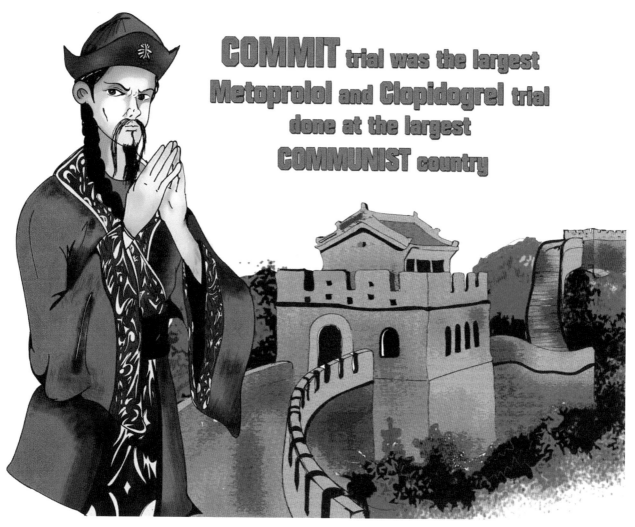

COMMIT trial was the largest Metoprolol and Clopidogrel trial done at the largest COMMUNIST country

COMMIT/CCS-2 TRIAL

Addition of clopidogrel to aspirin in 45,852 patients with acute myocardial infarction: randomised placebo-controlled trial. Chen ZM, et al. COMMIT (ClOpidogrel and Metoprolol in Myocardial Infarction Trial) collaborative group).

Lancet. 2005; November 5;366(9497):1607-21.

BACKGROUND

Despite improvements in the emergency treatment of myocardial infarction (MI), early mortality and morbidity remain high. The antiplatelet agent clopidogrel adds to the benefit of aspirin in acute coronary syndromes without ST-segment elevation, but its effects in patients with ST-elevation MI were unclear.

METHODS: 45,852 patients admitted to 1250 hospitals within 24 h of suspected acute MI onset were randomly allocated clopidogrel 75 mg daily (n=22,961) or matching placebo (n=22,891) in addition to aspirin 162 mg daily. 93% had ST-segment elevation or bundle branch block, and 7% had ST-segment depression. Treatment was to continue until discharge or up to 4 weeks in hospital (mean 15 days in survivors) and 93% of patients completed it. The two prespecified co-primary outcomes were: (1) the composite of death, reinfarction, or stroke; and (2) death from any cause during the scheduled treatment period. Comparisons were by intention to treat, and used the log-rank method. This trial is registered with ClinicalTrials.gov, number NCT00222573.

FINDINGS: Allocation to clopidogrel produced a highly significant 9% (95% CI 3-14) proportional reduction in death, reinfarction, or stroke (2121 [9.2%] clopidogrel vs 2310 [10.1%] placebo; p=0.002), corresponding to nine (SE 3) fewer events per 1000 patients treated for about 2 weeks. There was also a significant 7% (1-13) proportional reduction in any death (1726 [7.5%] vs 1845 [8.1%]; p=0.03). These effects on death, reinfarction, and stroke seemed consistent across a wide range of patients and independent of other treatments being used. Considering all fatal, transfused, or cerebral bleeds together, no significant excess risk was noted with clopidogrel, either overall (134 [0.58%] vs 125 [0.55%]; p=0.59), or in patients aged older than 70 years or in those given fibrinolytic therapy.

INTERPRETATION: In a wide range of patients with acute MI, adding clopidogrel 75 mg daily to aspirin and other standard treatments (such as fibrinolytic therapy) safely reduces mortality and major vascular events in hospital, and should be considered routinely.

Early intravenous then oral metoprolol in 45,852 patients with acute myocardial infarction: randomised placebo-controlled trial.

Chen ZM, et al. COMMIT (ClOpidogrel and Metoprolol in Myocardial Infarction Trial) collaborative group.

Lancet. 2005; November 5; 366(9497):1622-32.

BACKGROUND: Despite previous randomised trials of early beta-blocker therapy in the emergency treatment of myocardial infarction (MI), uncertainty has persisted about the value of adding it to current standard interventions (eg, aspirin and fibrinolytic therapy), and the balance of potential benefits and hazards is still unclear in high-risk patients.

METHODS: 45,852 patients admitted to 1250 hospitals within 24 h of suspected acute MI onset were randomly allocated metoprolol (up to 15 mg intravenous then 200 mg oral daily; n=22,929) or matching placebo (n=22,923). 93% had ST-segment elevation or bundle branch block, and 7% had ST-segment depression. Treatment was to continue until discharge or up to 4 weeks in hospital (mean 15 days in survivors) and 89% completed it. The two prespecified co-primary outcomes were: (1) composite of death, reinfarction, or cardiac arrest; and (2) death from any cause during the scheduled treatment period. Comparisons were by intention to treat, and used the log-rank method. This study is registered with ClinicalTrials.gov, number NCT 00222573.

FINDINGS: Neither of the co-primary outcomes was significantly reduced by allocation to metoprolol. For death, reinfarction, or cardiac arrest, 2166 (9.4%) patients allocated metoprolol had at least one such event compared with 2261 (9.9%) allocated placebo (odds ratio [OR] 0.96, 95% CI 0.90-1.01; p=0.1). For death alone, there were 1774 (7.7%) deaths in the metoprolol group versus 1797 (7.8%) in the placebo group (OR 0.99, 0.92-1.05; p=0.69). Allocation to metoprolol was associated with five fewer people having reinfarction (464 [2.0%] metoprolol vs 568 [2.5%] placebo; OR 0.82, 0.72-0.92; p=0.001) and five fewer having ventricular fibrillation (581 [2.5%] vs 698 [3.0%]; OR 0.83, 0.75-0.93; p=0.001) per 1000 treated. Overall, these reductions were counterbalanced by 11 more per 1000 developing cardiogenic shock (1141 [5.0%] vs 885 [3.9%]; OR 1.30, 1.19-1.41; p<0.00001). This excess of cardiogenic shock was mainly during days 0-1 after admission, whereas the reductions in reinfarction and ventricular fibrillation emerged more gradually. Consequently, the overall effect on death, reinfarction, arrest, or shock was significantly adverse during days 0-1 and significantly beneficial thereafter. There was substantial net hazard in haemodynamically unstable patients, and moderate net benefit in those who were relatively stable (particularly after days 0-1).

INTERPRETATION: The use of early beta-blocker therapy in acute MI reduces the risks of reinfarction and ventricular fibrillation, but increases the risk of cardiogenic shock, especially during the first day or so after admission. Consequently, it might generally be prudent to consider starting beta-blocker therapy in hospital only when the haemodynamic condition after MI has stabilised.

CLARITY-TIMI 28

Addition of Clopidogrel to Aspirin and Fibrinolytic Therapy for Myocardial Infarction with ST-Segment Elevation

Marc S.et al for the CLARITY-TIMI 28 Investigators

New England Journal of Medicine (NEJM) 2005; March 24, 352:1179-1189.

CLARITY trial showed the benefit of adding clopidogrel to aspirin and a standard fibrinolytic regimen, improving the patency rate of the infarct-related artery and reduces ischemic complications.

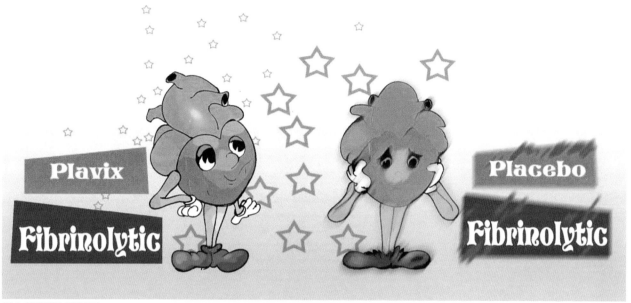

BACKGROUND

A substantial proportion of patients receiving fibrinolytic therapy for myocardial infarction with ST-segment elevation have inadequate reperfusion or reocclusion of the infarct-related artery, leading to an increased risk of complications and death.

METHODS

We enrolled 3491 patients, 18 to 75 years of age, who presented within 12 hours after the onset of an ST-elevation myocardial infarction and randomly assigned them to receive clopidogrel (300-mg loading dose, followed by 75 mg once daily) or placebo. Patients received a fibrinolytic agent, aspirin, and when appropriate, heparin (dispensed according to body weight) and were scheduled to undergo angiography 48 to 192 hours after the start of study medication. The primary efficacy end point was a composite of an occluded infarct-related artery (defined by a Thrombolysis in Myocardial Infarction flow grade of 0 or 1) on angiography or death or recurrent myocardial infarction before angiography.

RESULTS

The rates of the primary efficacy end point were 21.7 percent in the placebo group and 15.0 percent in the clopidogrel group, representing an absolute reduction of 6.7 percentage points in the rate and a 36 percent reduction in the odds of the end point with clopidogrel therapy (95 percent confidence interval, 24 to 47 percent; P<0.001). By 30 days, clopidogrel therapy reduced the odds of the composite end point of death from cardiovascular causes, recurrent myocardial infarction, or recurrent ischemia leading to the need for urgent revascularization by 20 percent (from 14.1 to 11.6 percent, P=0.03). The rates of major bleeding and intracranial hemorrhage were similar in the two groups.

CONCLUSIONS

In patients 75 years of age or younger who have myocardial infarction with ST-segment elevation and who receive aspirin and a standard fibrinolytic regimen, the addition of clopidogrel improves the patency rate of the infarct-related artery and reduces ischemic complications.

EXTRACT-TIMI 25 TRIAL

ENOXAPARIN VERSUS UNFRACTIONATED HEPARIN WITH FIBRINOLYSIS FOR ST-ELEVATION MYOCARDIAL INFARCTION.

NEW ENGLAND JOURNAL OF MEDICINE (NEJM) 2006.

The Enoxaparin (Lovenox) and fondaparinux are low molecular weight heparin, that were tested in ACS in EXTRACT and OASIS-5, OASIS-6 trials respectively.

EXTRACT trial was done to compare the low molecular heparin (Enoxaparin) to heparin in patients receiving fibrinolysis for ST-elevation myocardial infarction. It showed that Enoxaparin was superior to heparin but was associated with higher incident of major bleeding.

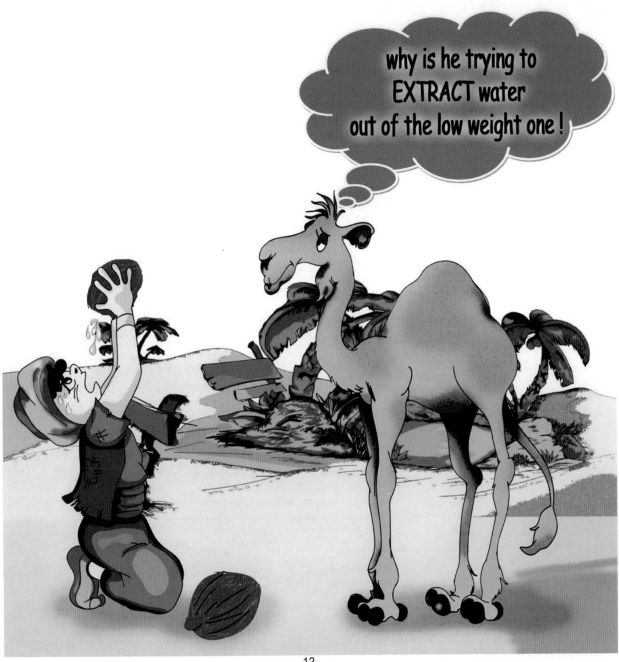

OASIS-5 AND OASIS-6 TRIALS

OASIS-5 compared Fonaparinux to Enoxaparin in the setting of acute coronary syndrome (ACS), while OASIS -6 compared Fonaparinux to UFH in the setting of STEMI.

As EXTRACT trial showed that Enoxaparin was effective in STEMI but was associated with increased risk bleeding. OASIS-5 trial was done to see whether fondaparinux would preserve the benefits of enoxaparin without the increase in the risk of bleeding, which was the case demonstrated in the results. Off note this study showed the difference in the setting in acute coronary syndrome in general, not only in STEMI like EXTRACT- 25 trial.

While OASIS-6 included only STEMI patients, Fonaparinux was compared to UFH. The primary outcome was the composite of death or reinfarction at 30 days. There was a reduction in the primary outcome between the 2 groups. That was mainly observed in those who received thrombolytic therapy and those not receiving any reperfusion therapy, but not in the ones who underwent primary percutaneous coronary intervention.

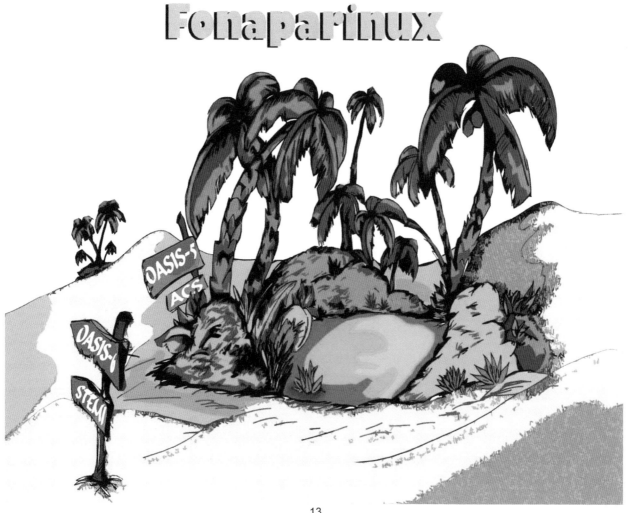

ExTRACT-TIMI 25 TRIAL

Enoxaparin versus Unfractionated Heparin with Fibrinolysis for ST-Elevation Myocardial Infarction.

Elliott M. Antman et al. for the ExTRACT-TIMI 25 Investigators

New England Journal of Medicine (NEJM) 2006; April 6;354:1477-1488

BACKGROUND

Unfractionated heparin is often used as adjunctive therapy with fibrinolysis in patients with ST-elevation myocardial infarction. We compared a low-molecular-weight heparin, enoxaparin, with unfractionated heparin for this purpose.

METHODS

We randomly assigned 20,506 patients with ST-elevation myocardial infarction who were scheduled to undergo fibrinolysis to receive enoxaparin throughout the index hospitalization or weight-based unfractionated heparin for at least 48 hours. The primary efficacy end point was death or nonfatal recurrent myocardial infarction through 30 days.

RESULTS

The primary end point occurred in 12.0 percent of patients in the unfractionated heparin group and 9.9 percent of those in the enoxaparin group (17 percent reduction in relative risk, P<0.001). Nonfatal reinfarction occurred in 4.5 percent of the patients receiving unfractionated heparin and 3.0 percent of those receiving enoxaparin (33 percent reduction in relative risk, P<0.001); 7.5 percent of patients given unfractionated heparin died, as did 6.9 percent of those given enoxaparin (P = 0.11). The composite of death, nonfatal reinfarction, or urgent revascularization occurred in 14.5 percent of patients given unfractionated heparin and 11.7 percent of those given enoxaparin (P<0.001); major bleeding occurred in 1.4 percent and 2.1 percent, respectively (P<0.001). The composite of death, nonfatal reinfarction, or nonfatal intracranial hemorrhage (a measure of net clinical benefit) occurred in 12.2 percent of patients given unfractionated heparin and 10.1 percent of those given enoxaparin (P<0.001).

CONCLUSIONS

In patients receiving fibrinolysis for ST-elevation myocardial infarction, treatment with enoxaparin throughout the index hospitalization is superior to treatment with unfractionated heparin for 48 hours but is associated with an increase in major bleeding episodes. These findings should be interpreted in the context of net clinical benefit.

OASIS 5

Comparison of Fondaparinux and Enoxaparin in Acute Coronary Syndromes

The Fifth Organization to Assess Strategies in Acute Ischemic Syndromes Investigators*

New England Journal of Medicine (NEJM) 2006; April 6; 354:1464-1476.

BACKGROUND

The combined use of anticoagulants, antiplatelet agents, and invasive coronary procedures reduces ischemic coronary events but also increases bleeding in patients with acute coronary syndromes. We therefore assessed whether fondaparinux would preserve the anti-ischemic benefits of enoxaparin while reducing bleeding.

METHODS

We randomly assigned 20,078 patients with acute coronary syndromes to receive either fondaparinux (2.5 mg daily) or enoxaparin (1 mg per kilogram of body weight twice daily) for a mean of six days and evaluated death, myocardial infarction, or refractory ischemia at nine days (the primary outcome); major bleeding; and their combination. Patients were followed for up to sixmonths.

RESULTS

The number of patients with primary-outcome events was similar in the two groups (579 with fondaparinux [5.8 percent] vs. 573 with enoxaparin [5.7 percent]; hazard ratio in the fondaparinux group, 1.01; 95 percent confidence interval, 0.90 to 1.13), satisfying the noninferiority criteria. The number of events meeting this combined outcome showed a nonsignificant trend toward a lower value in the fondaparinux group at 30 days (805 vs. 864, P = 0.13) and at the end of the study (1222 vs. 1308, P = 0.06). The rate of major bleeding at nine days was markedly lower with fon daparinux than with enoxaparin (217 events [2.2 percent] vs. 412 events [4.1 percent]; hazard ratio, 0.52; P<0.001). The composite of the primary outcome and major bleeding at nine days favored fondaparinux (737 events [7.3 percent] vs. 905 events [9.0 percent]; hazard ratio, 0.81; P<0.001). Fondaparinux was associated with a significantly reduced number of deaths at 30 days (295 vs. 352, P = 0.02) and at 180 days (574 vs. 638, P = 0.05).

CONCLUSION

Fondaparinux is similar to enoxaparin in reducing the risk of ischemic events at nine days, but it substantially reduces major bleeding and improves long term mortality and morbidity.

OASIS-6 Trial

Effects of fondaparinux on mortality and reinfarction in patients with acute ST-segment elevation myocardial infarction: the OASIS-6 randomized trial.

Yusuf S, et al.

Journal of the American Medical Association (JAMA)   2006 ; April 5; 295(13):1519-30.

CONTEXT

Despite many therapeutic advances, mortality in patients with acute ST-segment elevation myocardial infarction (STEMI) remains high. The role of additional antithrombotic agents is unclear, especially among patients not receiving reperfusion therapy.

OBJECTIVE

To evaluate the effect of fondaparinux, a factor Xa inhibitor, when initiated early and given for up to 8 days vs usual care (placebo in those in whom unfractionated heparin [UFH] is not indicated [stratum 1] or unfractionated heparin for up to 48 hours followed by placebo for up to 8 days [stratum 2]) in patients with STEMI.

DESIGN, SETTING, AND PARTICIPANTS:

Randomized double-blind comparison of fondaparinux 2.5 mg once daily or control for up to 8 days in 12,092 patients with STEMI from 447 hospitals in 41 countries (September 2003-January 2006). From day 3 through day 9, all patients received either fondaparinux or placebo according to the original randomized assignment.

MAIN OUTCOME MEASURES:

Composite of death or reinfarction at 30 days (primary) with secondary assessments at 9 days and at final follow-up (3 or 6 months).

RESULTS

Death or reinfarction at 30 days was significantly reduced from 677 (11.2%) of 6056 patients in the control group to 585 (9.7%) of 6036 patients in the fondaparinux group (hazard ratio [HR], 0.86; 95% confidence interval [CI], 0.77-0.96; $P = .008$); absolute risk reduction, 1.5%; 95% CI, 0.4%-2.6%). These benefits were observed at 9 days (537 [8.9%] placebo vs 444 [7.4%] fondaparinux; HR, 0.83; 95% CI, 0.73-0.94; $P = .003$, and at study end (857 [14.8%] placebo vs 756 [13.4%] fondaparinux; HR, 0.88; 95% CI, 0.79-0.97; $P = .008$). Mortality was significantly reduced throughout the study. There was no heterogeneity of the effects of fondaparinux in the 2 strata by planned heparin use. However, there was no benefit in those undergoing primary percutaneous coronary intervention. In other patients in stratum 2, fondaparinux was superior to unfractionated heparin in preventing death or reinfarction at 30 days (HR, 0.82; 95% CI, 0.66-1.02; $P = .08$) and at study end (HR, 0.77; 95% CI, 0.64-0.93; $P = .008$). Significant benefits were observed in those receiving thrombolytic therapy (HR, 0.79; $P = .003$) and those not receiving any reperfusion therapy (HR, 0.80; $P = .03$). There was a tendency to fewer severe bleeds (79 for placebo vs 61 for fondaparinux; $P = .13$), with significantly fewer cardiac tamponade (48 vs 28; $P = .02$) with fondaparinux at 9 days.

CONCLUSION

In patients with STEMI, particularly those not undergoing primary percutaneous coronary intervention, fondaparinux significantly reduces mortality and reinfarction without increasing bleeding and strokes.

PLATO TRIAL

TICAGRELOR VERSUS CLOPIDOGREL IN PATIENTS WITH ACUTE CORONARY SYNDROMES.
NEW ENGLAND JOURNAL OF MEDICINE (NEJM) 2009.

This study tried to compare Ticagrelor is an oral, reversible, direct-acting inhibitor of the adenosine diphosphate receptor P2Y12, with clopidogrel in the setting of acute coronary syndrome , with or without ST-segment elevation. The primary end point was a composite of death from vascular causes, myocardial infarction, or stroke. Results showed that treatment with ticagrelor as compared with clopidogrel significantly reduced the rate of death from vascular causes, myocardial infarction, or stroke without an increase in the rate of overall major bleeding but with an increase in the rate of non–procedure-related bleeding.

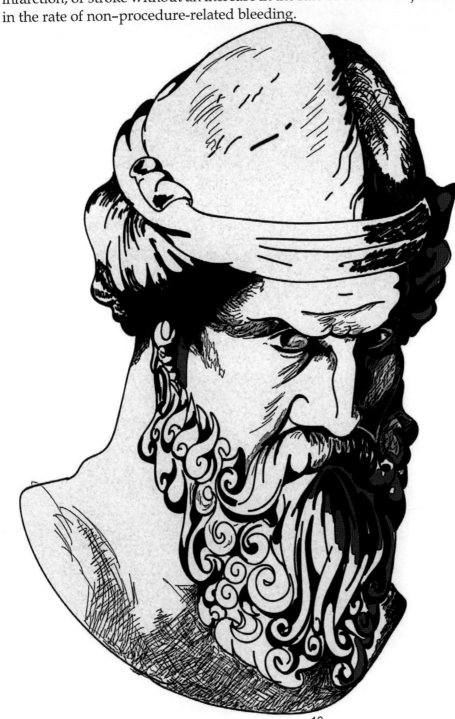

Ticagrelor
clopidogrel

PLATO TRIAL

Ticagrelor versus clopidogrel in patients with acute coronary syndromes.

Wallentin L et al

New England Journal of Medicine (NEJM) 2009; September 10; 361(11):1045-57

BACKGROUND

Ticagrelor is an oral, reversible, direct-acting inhibitor of the adenosine diphosphate receptor P2Y12 that has a more rapid onset and more pronounced platelet inhibition than clopidogrel.

METHODS

In this multicenter, double-blind, randomized trial, we compared ticagrelor (180-mg loading dose, 90 mg twice daily thereafter) and clopidogrel (300-to-600-mg loading dose, 75 mg daily thereafter) for the prevention of cardiovascular events in 18,624 patients admitted to the hospital with an acute coronary syndrome, with or without ST-segment elevation.

RESULTS

At 12 months, the primary end point--a composite of death from vascular causes, myocardial infarction, or stroke--had occurred in 9.8% of patients receiving ticagrelor as compared with 11.7% of those receiving clopidogrel (hazard ratio, 0.84; 95% confidence interval [CI], 0.77 to 0.92; P<0.001). Predefined hierarchical testing of secondary end points showed significant differences in the rates of other composite end points, as well as myocardial infarction alone (5.8% in the ticagrelor group vs. 6.9% in the clopidogrel group, P=0.005) and death from vascular causes (4.0% vs. 5.1%, P=0.001) but not stroke alone (1.5% vs. 1.3%, P=0.22). The rate of death from any cause was also reduced with ticagrelor (4.5%, vs. 5.9% with clopidogrel; P<0.001). No significant difference in the rates of major bleeding was found between the ticagrelor and clopidogrel groups (11.6% and 11.2%, respectively; P=0.43), but ticagrelor was associated with a higher rate of major bleeding not related to coronary-artery bypass grafting (4.5% vs. 3.8%, P=0.03), including more instances of fatal intracranial bleeding and fewer of fatal bleeding of other types.

CONCLUSIONS

In patients who have an acute coronary syndrome with or without ST-segment elevation, treatment with ticagrelor as compared with clopidogrel significantly reduced the rate of death from vascular causes, myocardial infarction, or stroke without an increase in the rate of overall major bleeding but with an increase in the rate of non-procedure-related bleeding.

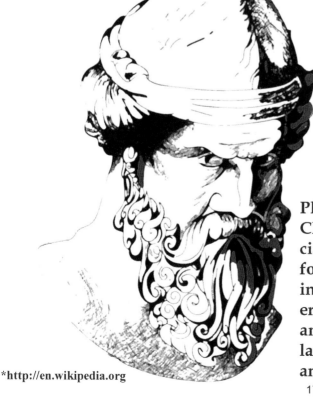

Plato (429- 347 BC) was a philosopher in Classical Greece. He was also a mathematician, writer of philosophical dialogues, and founder of the Academy in Athens, the first institution of higher learning in the Western world. Along with his mentor, Socrates, and his student, Aristotle, Plato helped to lay the foundations of Western philosophy and science*.

*http://en.wikipedia.org

ADMIRAL AND CADILLAC TRAILS

These two trials were one of the earliest evaluating GPIIb/IIIa in acute MI. In ADMIRAL trial the abciximab (ReoPro) was administered to patient with acute ST elevation myocardial infarct prior to arrival to the cath lab, while in the CADILLAC trial the abciximab was administered during the PTCA/Stenting procedure. The ADMIRAL showed that early administration of abciximab in patients with acute myocardial infarction improves coronary patency, the success rate of the stenting procedure, the rate of coronary patency at six months, left ventricular function, and clinical outcomes.

While in the CADILLAC trial patients with acute myocardial infarction were randomized to one of the following groups; 1) balloon angioplasty alone, 2) balloon angioplasty plus abciximab, 3) stenting alone, or 4) stenting plus abciximab. And it showed that the event-free survival was greatest in patients assigned to routine stenting (with or without abciximab), intermediate in patients assigned to PTCA plus abciximab, and lowest in those assigned to PTCA only.

The Cadillac Admiral
Abciximab

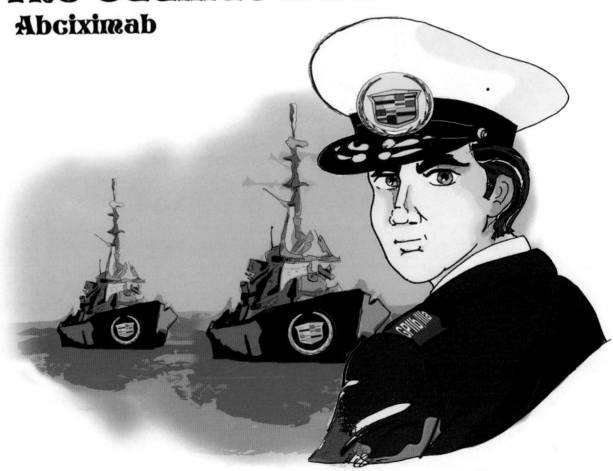

ADMIRAL TRAIL

Platelet glycoprotein IIb/IIIa inhibition with coronary stenting for acute myocardial infarction. Montalescot G, et al. ADMIRAL Investigators..

New England Journal of Medicine (NEJM). 2001; June 21; 344(25):1895-903.

BACKGROUND

When administered in conjunction with primary coronary stenting for the treatment of acute myocardial infarction, a platelet glycoprotein IIb/IIIa inhibitor may provide additional clinical benefit, but data on this combination therapy are limited.

METHODS

We randomly assigned 300 patients with acute myocardial infarction in a double-blind fashion either to abciximab plus stenting (149 patients) or placebo plus stenting (151 patients) before they underwent coronary angiography. Clinical outcomes were evaluated 30 days and 6 months after the procedure. The angiographic patency of the infarct-related vessel and the left ventricular ejection fraction were evaluated at 24 hours and 6 months.

RESULTS

At 30 days, the primary end point--a composite of death, reinfarction, or urgent revascularization of the target vessel--had occurred in 6.0 percent of the patients in the abciximab group, as compared with 14.6 percent of those in the placebo group (P=0.01); at 6 months, the corresponding figures were 7.4 percent and 15.9 percent (P=0.02). The better clinical outcomes in the abciximab group were related to the greater frequency of grade 3 coronary flow (according to the classification of the Thrombolysis in Myocardial Infarction trial) in this group than in the placebo group before the procedure (16.8 percent vs. 5.4 percent, P=0.01), immediately afterward (95.1 percent vs. 86.7 percent, P=0.04), and six months afterward (94.3 percent vs. 82.8 percent, P=0.04). One major bleeding event occurred in the abciximab group (0.7 percent); none occurred in the placebo group.

CONCLUSIONS

As compared with placebo, early administration of abciximab in patients with acute myocardial infarction improves coronary patency before stenting, the success rate of the stenting procedure, the rate of coronary patency at six months, left ventricular function, and clinical outcomes.

CADILLAC TRIAL

Comparison of angioplasty with stenting, with or without abciximab, in acute myocardial infarction. Stone GW, et al.

New England Journal of Medicine (NEJM). 2002; March; 28; 346(13):957-66

BACKGROUND

As compared with thrombolytic therapy, primary percutaneous transluminal coronary angioplasty (PTCA) in acute myocardial infarction reduces the rates of death, reinfarction, and stroke, but recurrent ischemia, restenosis, and reocclusion of the infarct-related artery remain problematic. When used in combination with PTCA, coronary stenting and platelet glycoprotein IIb/IIIa inhibitors may further improve outcomes.

METHODS

Using a 2-by-2 factorial design, we randomly assigned 2082 patients with acute myocardial infarction to undergo PTCA alone (518 patients), PTCA plus abciximab therapy (528), stenting alone with the MultiLink stent (512), or stenting plus abciximab therapy (524).

RESULTS

Normal flow was restored in the target vessel in 94.5 to 96.9 percent of patients and did not vary according to the reperfusion strategy. At six months, the primary end point - a composite of death, reinfarction, disabling stroke, and ischemia-driven revascularization of the target vessel - had occurred in 20.0 percent of patients after PTCA, 16.5 percent after PTCA plus abciximab, 11.5 percent after stenting, and 10.2 percent afterstenting plus abciximab (P<0.001). There were no significant differences among the groups in the rates of death, stroke, or reinfarction; the difference in the incidence of the primary end point was due entirely to differences in the rates of target-vessel revascularization (ranging from 15.7 percent after PTCA to 5.2 percent after stenting plus abciximab, P<0.001). The rate of angiographically established restenosis was 40.8 percent after PTCA and 22.2 percent after stenting (P<0.001), and the respective rates of reocclusion of the infarcted-related artery were 11.3 percent and 5.7 percent (P=0.01), both independent of abciximab use.

CONCLUSIONS

At experienced centers, stent implantation (with or without abciximab therapy) should be considered the routine reperfusion strategy.

BRAVE-3 AND ISAR-REACT 2 TRIALS

In patients with acute STEMI undergoing primary PCI after pretreatment with a 600 mg loading dose of clopidogrel, the additional use of abciximab (ReoPro) is not associated with further reduction in infarct size. In contrary to ISAR-REACT 2 trial showed benefit of the glycoprotein IIb/IIIa inhibitor abciximab in patients with non-ST-segment elevation acute coronary syndromes (ACS) undergoing percutaneous coronary intervention (PCI) after pretreatment with 600 mg of clopidogrel.

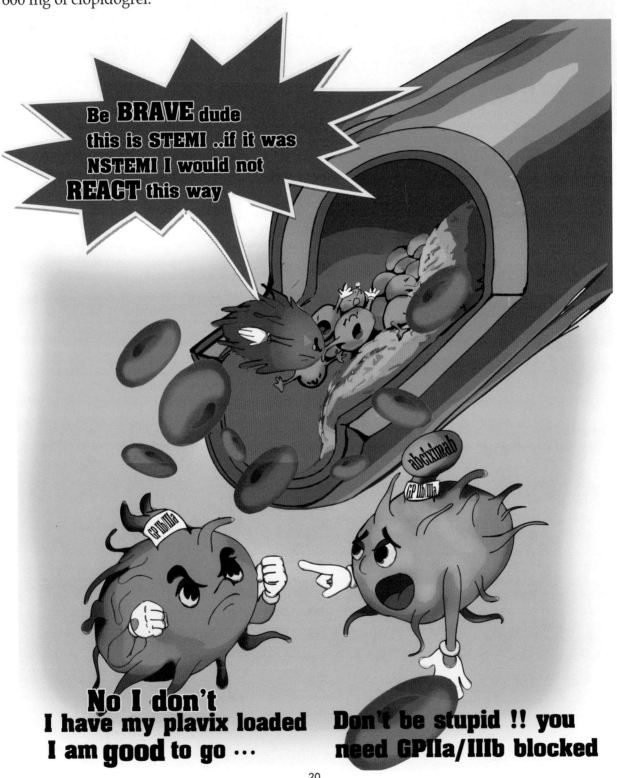

BRAVE-3 TRIAL

Abciximab in patients with acute ST-segment-elevation myocardial infarction undergoing primary percutaneous coronary intervention after clopidogrel loading: a randomized double-blind trial.

Mehilli J et al. Bavarian Reperfusion Alternatives Evaluation-3 (BRAVE-3) Study Investigators.
Circulation. 2009; April 14; 119(14):1933-40.

BACKGROUND

The glycoprotein IIb/IIIa receptor inhibitor abciximab has improved the efficacy of primary percutaneous coronary interventions in patients with acute myocardial infarction. However, it is not known whether abciximab remains beneficial after adequate clopidogrel loading in patients with acute ST-segment-elevation myocardial infarction.

METHODS AND RESULTS

A total of 800 patients with acute ST-segment-elevation myocardial infarction within 24 hours from symptom onset, all treated with 600 mg clopidogrel, were randomly assigned in a double-blind fashion to receive either abciximab (n=401) or placebo (n=399) in the intensive care unit before being sent to the catheterization laboratory. The primary end point, infarct size measured by single-photon emission computed tomography with technetium-99m sestamibi before hospital discharge, was 15.7+/-17.2% (mean+/-SD) of the left ventricle in the abciximab group and 16.6+/-18.6% of the left ventricle in the placebo group (P=0.47). At 30 days, the composite of death, recurrent myocardial infarction, stroke, or urgent revascularization of the infarct-related artery was observed in 20 patients in the abciximab group (5.0%) and 15 patients in the placebo group (3.8%) (relative risk, 1.3; 95% CI, 0.7 to 2.6; P=0.40). Major bleeding complications were observed in 7 patients in each group (1.8%).

CONCLUSIONS

Upstream administration of abciximab is not associated with a reduction in infarct size in patients presenting with acute myocardial infarction within 24 hours of symptom onset and receiving 600 mg clopidogrel.

ISAR-REACT 2

Abciximab in patients with acute coronary syndromes undergoing percutaneous coronary intervention after clopidogrel pretreatment: the ISAR-REACT 2 randomized trial. Kastrati A et al.

Journal of the American Medical Association (JAMA) 2006, April 5; 295(13):1531-8

CONTEXT No specifically designed studies have addressed the role of the glycoprotein IIb/IIIa inhibitor abciximab in patients with non-ST-segment elevation acute coronary syndromes (ACS) undergoing percutaneous coronary intervention (PCI) after pretreatment with 600 mg of clopidogrel.

OBJECTIVE To assess whether abciximab is associated with clinical benefit in high-risk patients with ACS undergoing PCI after pretreatment with 600 mg of clopidogrel.

DESIGN, SETTING, AND PATIENTS

International, multicenter, randomized, double-blind, placebo-controlled study conducted from March 2003 through December 2005, enrolling 2022 patients (mean age, 66 years) with non-ST-segment elevation ACS undergoing PCI.

INTERVENTIONS: Patients were assigned to receive either abciximab (0.25 mg/kg of body weight bolus, followed by a 0.125-microg/kg per minute [maximum, 10 microg/min] infusion for 12 hours, plus heparin, 70 U/kg of body weight) or placebo (placebo bolus and infusion of 12 hours, plus heparin bolus, 140 U/kg). All patients received clopidogrel, 600 mg, at least 2 hours prior to the procedure, as well as 500 mg of oral or intravenous aspirin.

MAIN OUTCOME MEASURES: The primary end point was a composite of death, myocardial infarction, or urgent target vessel revascularization occurring within 30 days after randomization; secondary end points were rates of in-hospital major and minor bleeding.

RESULTS: Of 2022 patients enrolled, 1012 were assigned to abciximab and 1010 to placebo. The primary end point was reached in 90 patients (8.9%) assigned to abciximab vs 120 patients (11.9%) assigned to placebo, a 25% reduction in risk with abciximab (relative risk [RR], 0.75; 95% CI, 0.58-0.97; P = .03). Among patients without an elevated troponin level, there was no difference in the incidence of primary end point events between the abciximab group (23/499 patients [4.6%]) and the placebo group (22/474 patients [4.6%]) (RR, 0.99; 95% CI, 0.56-1.76; P = .98), whereas among patients with an elevated troponin level, the incidence of events was significantly lower in the abciximab group (67/513 patients [13.1%]) compared with the placebo group (98/536 patients [18.3%]), which corresponds to an RR of 0.71 (95% CI, 0.54-0.95; P = .02) (P = .07 for interaction). There were no significant differences between the 2 groups regarding the risk of major and minor bleeding as well as need for transfusion.

CONCLUSIONS: Abciximab reduces the risk of adverse events in patients with non-ST-segment elevation ACS undergoing PCI after pretreatment with 600 mg of clopidogrel. The benefits provided by abciximab appear to be confined to patients presenting with an elevated troponin level.

ON TIME-2 TRIAL

PREHOSPITAL INITIATION OF TIROFIBAN IN PATIENTS WITH ST-ELEVATION MYOCARDIAL INFARCTION UNDERGOING PRIMARY ANGIOPLASTY (ON-TIME 2)
LANCET. 2008.

This trial showed that the routine prehospital initiation of high-bolus dose glycoprotein IIb/IIIa blocker tirofiban improved ST-segment resolution and clinical outcome after PCI, emphasizes that further platelet aggregation inhibition besides high-dose clopidogrel is mandated in patients with STEMI undergoing PCI.

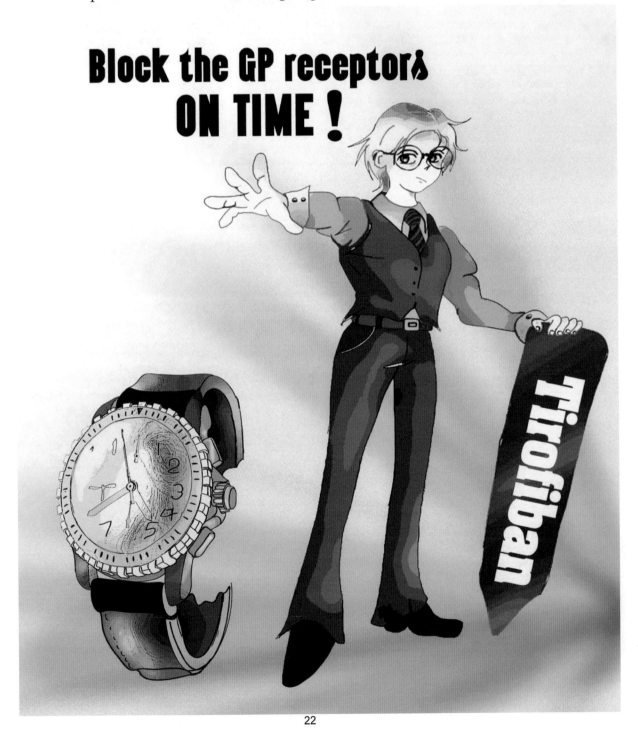

On time-2 TRIAL

Prehospital initiation of tirofiban in patients with ST-elevation myocardial infarction undergoing primary angioplasty (On-TIME 2): a multicentre, double-blind, randomised controlled trial. Van't Hof AW et al.

Lancet. 2008; August 16; 372(9638):537-46

BACKGROUND

The most effective magnitude and timing of antiplatelet therapy is important in patients with acute ST-elevation myocardial infarction (STEMI). We investigated whether the results of primary coronary angioplasty (PCI) can be improved by the early administration of the glycoprotein IIb/IIIa blocker tirofiban at first medical contact in the ambulance or referral centre.

METHODS

We undertook a double-blind, randomised, placebo-controlled trial in 24 centres in the Netherlands, Germany, and Belgium. Between June 29, 2006, and Nov 13, 2007, 984 patients with STEMI who were candidates to undergo PCI were randomly assigned to either high-bolus dose tirofiban (n=491) or placebo (N=493) in addition to aspirin (500 mg), heparin (5000 IU), and clopidogrel (600 mg). Randomisation was by blinded sealed kits with study drug, in blocks of four. The primary endpoint was the extent of residual ST-segment deviation 1 h after PCI. Analysis was by intention to treat. The trial is registered, number ISRCTN06195297.

FINDINGS

936 (95%) patients were randomly assigned to treatment after a prehospital diagnosis of myocardial infarction in the ambulance. Median time from onset of symptoms to diagnosis was 76 min (IQR 35-150). Mean residual ST deviation before PCI (10.9 mm [SD 9.2] vs 12.1 mm [9.4], p=0.028) and 1 h after PCI (3.6 mm [4.6] vs 4.8 mm [6.3], p=0.003) was significantly lower in patients pretreated with high-bolus dose tirofiban than in those assigned to placebo. The rate of major bleeding did not differ significantly between the two groups (19 [4%] vs 14 [3%]; p=0.36).

INTERPRETATION

Our finding that routine prehospital initiation of high-bolus dose tirofiban improved ST-segment resolution and clinical outcome after PCI, emphasises that further platelet aggregation inhibition besides high-dose clopidogrel is mandated in patients with STEMI undergoing PCI.

HORIZONS-AMI TRIAL

BIVALIRUDIN DURING PRIMARY PCI IN ACUTE MYOCARDIAL INFARCTION.
NEW ENGLAND JOURNAL OF MEDICINE (NEJM) 2008.

This trial compared the direct thrombin inhibitor (bivalirudin) to heparin plus glycoprotein IIb/IIIa inhibitors in patients with STEMI undergoing primary PCI. Bivalirudin group had lower 30 days of bleeding\ complications, and lower rate of mortality. Albeit there was an increase in the acute stent thrombosis within 24 hours in the bivalirudin group.

UFH+GP IIb/IIIa inhibitors vs Bivalirudin

HORIZONS-AMI TRIAL

Bivalirudin during primary PCI in acute myocardial infarction.

Stone GW et al. HORIZONS-AMI Trial Investigators.

New England Journal of Medicine (NEJM) 2008; May 22; 358(21):2218-30

BACKGROUND

Treatment with the direct thrombin inhibitor bivalirudin, as compared with heparin plus glycoprotein IIb/IIIa inhibitors, results in similar suppression of ischemia while reducing hemorrhagic complications in patients with stable angina and non-ST-segment elevation acute coronary syndromes who are undergoing percutaneous coronary intervention (PCI). The safety and efficacy of bivalirudin in high-risk patients are unknown.

METHODS

We randomly assigned 3602 patients with ST-segment elevation myocardial infarction who presented within 12 hours after the onset of symptoms and who were undergoing primary PCI to treatment with heparin plus a glycoprotein IIb/IIIa inhibitor or to treatment with bivalirudin alone. The two primary end points of the study were major bleeding and combined adverse clinical events, defined as the combination of major bleeding or major adverse cardiovascular events, including death, reinfarction, target-vessel revascularization for ischemia, and stroke (hereinafter referred to as net adverse clinical events) within 30 days.

RESULTS

Anticoagulation with bivalirudin alone, as compared with heparin plus glycoprotein IIb/IIIa inhibitors, resulted in a reduced 30-day rate of net adverse clinical events (9.2% v_s. 12.1%; relative risk, 0.76; 95% confidence interval [CI] 0.63 to 0.92; P=0.005), owing to a lower rate of major bleeding (4.9% vs. 8.3%; relative risk, 0.60; 95% CI, 0.46 to 0.77; P<0.001). There was an increased risk of acute stent thrombosis within 24 hours in the bivalirudin group, but no significant increase was present by 30 days. Treatment with bivalirudin alone, as compared with heparin plus glycoprotein IIb/IIIa inhibitors, resulted in significantly lower 30-day rates of death from cardiac causes (1.8% vs. 2.9%; relative risk, 0.62; 95% CI, 0.40 to 0.95; P=0.03) and death from all causes (2.1% vs. 3.1%; relative risk, 0.66; 95% CI, 0.44 to 1.00; P=0.047).

CONCLUSIONS

In patients with ST-segment elevation myocardial infarction who are undergoing primary PCI, anticoagulation with bivalirudin alone, as compared with heparin plus glycoprotein IIb/IIIa inhibitors, results in significantly reduced 30-day rates of major bleeding and net adverse clinical events.

REACT TRIAL

RESCUE ANGIOPLASTY AFTER FAILED THROMBOLYTIC THERAPY FOR ACUTE MYOCARDIAL INFARCTION.
NEW ENGLAND JOURNAL OF MEDICINE (NEJM) 2005.

REACT trial looked at what is the optimal strategy to follow if reperfusion fails to occur after thrombolytic therapy for acute myocardial infarction. Event-free survival after failed thrombolytic therapy was significantly higher with rescue PCI than with repeated thrombolysis or conservative treatment. Rescue PCI should be considered for patients in whom reperfusion fails to occur after thrombolytic therapy.

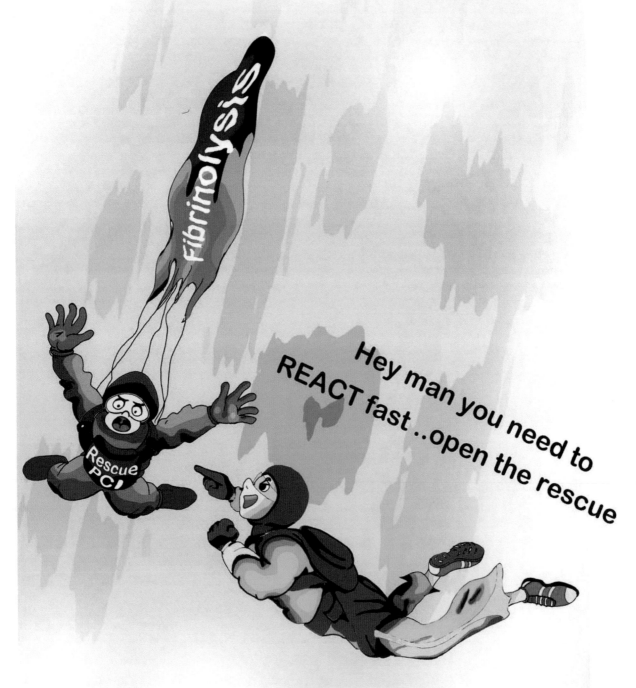

REACT Trial

Rescue angioplasty after failed thrombolytic therapy for acute myocardial infarction.

Gershlick AH et al.

New England Journal of Medicine (NEJM) 2005; December 29; 353(26):2758-68.

BACKGROUND

The appropriate treatment for patients in whom reperfusion fails to occur after thrombolytic therapy for acute myocardial infarction remains unclear. There are few data comparing emergency percutaneous coronary intervention (rescue PCI) with conservative care in such patients, and none comparing rescue PCI with repeated thrombolysis.

METHODS

We conducted a multicenter trial in the United Kingdom involving 427 patients with ST-segment elevation myocardial infarction in whom reperfusion failed to occur (less than 50 percent ST-segment resolution) within 90 minutes after thrombolytic treatment. The patients were randomly assigned to repeated thrombolysis (142 patients), conservative treatment (141 patients), or rescue PCI (144 patients). The primary end point was a composite of death, reinfarction, stroke, or severe heart failure within six months.

RESULTS

The rate of event-free survival among patients treated with rescue PCI was 84.6 percent, as compared with 70.1 percent among those receiving conservative therapy and 68.7 percent among those undergoing repeated thrombolysis (overall P=0.004). The adjusted hazard ratio for the occurrence of the primary end point for repeated thrombolysis versus conservative therapy was 1.09 (95 percent confidence interval, 0.71 to 1.67; P=0.69), as compared with adjusted hazard ratios of 0.43 (95 percent confidence interval, 0.26 to 0.72; P=0.001) for rescue PCI versus repeated thrombolysis and 0.47 (95 percent confidence interval, 0.28 to 0.79; P=0.004) for rescue PCI versus conservative therapy. There were no significant differences in mortality from all causes. Nonfatal bleeding, mostly at the sheath-insertion site, was more common with rescue PCI. At six months, 86.2 percent of the rescue-PCI group were free from revascularization, as compared with 77.6 percent of the conservative-therapy group and 74.4 percent of the repeated-thrombolysis group (overall P=0.05).

CONCLUSIONS

Event-free survival after failed thrombolytic therapy was significantly higher with rescue PCI than with repeated thrombolysis or conservative treatment. Rescue PCI should be considered for patients in whom reperfusion fails to occur after thrombolytic therapy.

FINESSE AND ASSENT-4 PCI TRIALS

Facilitating PCI is a pharmacological pretreatment with thrombolysis as an attempt to open the affected vessel prior to PCI. The FINESS and the ASSENT-4 trials evaluated whether patients with ST-segment elevation MI, who are expected to have a delay until catheterization would benefit from facilitated PCI with reduced-dose reteplase abciximab or abciximab alone vs. palcebo (FINESS) or with a full-dose tenecteplase (ASSENT-4). However Results showed no significant difference between pretreatment or placebo groups in the FINESS trial, while full-dose tenecteplase in ASSENT-4 was associated with more major adverse events than PCI alone in STEMI and cannot be recommended.

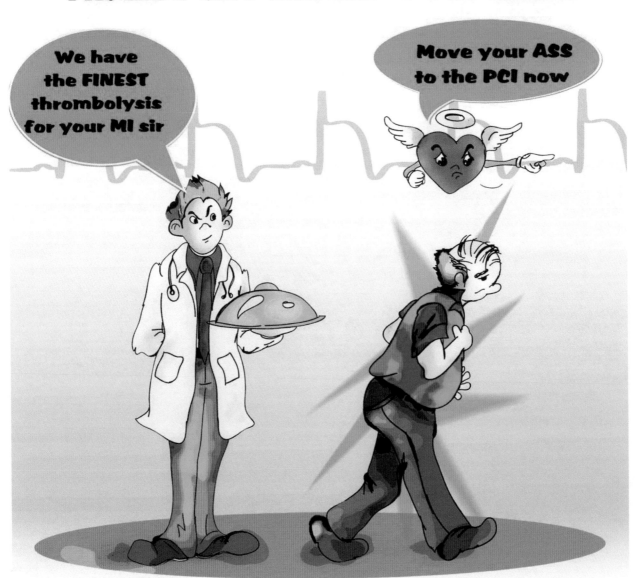

FINESSE TRIAL

1-YEAR SURVIVAL IN A RANDOMIZED TRIAL OF FACILITATED REPERFUSION: RESULTS FROM THE FINESSE (FACILITATED INTERVENTION WITH ENHANCED REPERFUSION SPEED TO STOP EVENTS) TRIAL. ELLIS SG ET AL.

Journal of the American College of Cardiology (JACC)2009; October2; (10):909-16.

OBJECTIVES:

The aim of this report was to evaluate 12-month outcomes of facilitated percutaneous coronary intervention (PCI) in the FINESSE (Facilitated Intervention with Enhanced Reperfusion Speed to Stop Events) trial.

BACKGROUND:

Treatment delays remain common for patients with primary PCI leading to studies evaluating possible benefit of "facilitated" PCI. In the FINESSE trial, no reduction in the 90-day primary ischemic end point and an increase in bleeding were observed with both facilitated approaches, although modest favorable trends were seen for some patient subgroups.

METHODS:

A total of 2,452 patients with ST-segment elevation myocardial infarction (MI) and anticipated 1 to 4 h delay until catheterization were randomized to reduced-dose reteplase + abciximab, abciximab alone, or placebo, followed by expedited primary PCI. Placebo-treated patients received abciximab in the cath lab. One-year mortality was a pre-specified secondary end point.

RESULTS:

One-year mortalities in the 3 groups noted in the preceding text were 6.3%, 7.4%, and 7.0%, respectively (p = NS), representing 1.1%, 1.9%, and 2.5% increments since the 90-day outcome (p = 0.053 for combination treatment vs. primary PCI). A favorable trend with combination treatment was seen for patients with anterior MI (p = 0.09), but no other specified groups benefited or tended to benefit. Independent baseline correlates of 1-year mortality were systolic blood pressure <100 mm Hg, prior MI, age, Killip class >1, anterior MI, body mass index < or =25 kg/m(2), heart rate >100 beats/min, and no statin use.

CONCLUSIONS:

These results suggest that widespread utilization of the facilitated approaches tested cannot be justified, but that high-risk patient groups such as patients with anterior MI may deserve further study

ASSENT-4 PCI

PRIMARY VERSUS TENECTEPLASE-FACILITATED PERCUTANEOUS CORONARY INTERVENTION IN PATIENTS WITH ST-SEGMENT ELEVATION ACUTE MYOCARDIAL INFARCTION (ASSENT-4 PCI): RANDOMISED TRIAL.

Lancet. 2006 February 18; 367(9510):569-78.

BACKGROUND: Primary percutaneous coronary intervention (PCI) is more effective than fibrinolytic therapy for ST-segment elevation acute myocardial infarction (STEMI), but time to intervention can be considerable. Our aim was to investigate whether the administration of full-dose tenecteplase before a delayed PCI could mitigate the negative effect of this delay.

METHODS:

We did a randomised study in which we assigned patients with STEMI of less than 6 h duration (scheduled to undergo primary PCI with an anticipated delay of 1-3 h) to standard PCI (n=838) or PCI preceded by administration of full-dose tenecteplase (n=829). All patients received aspirin and a bolus, without an infusion, of unfractionated heparin. Our primary endpoint was death or congestive heart failure or shock within 90 days. Analyses were by intention to treat. This study is registered with , number NCT00168792.

FINDINGS:

We planned to enroll 4000 patients, but early cessation of enrollment was recommended by the data and safety monitoring board because of a higher in-hospital mortality in the facilitated than in the standard PCI group (6% [43 of 664] vs 3% [22 of 656], p=0.0105). Of those enrolled, six were lost to follow-up in the facilitated PCI group and seven in the other group. Median time from randomisation to first balloon inflation was similar in both groups. The median time from bolus tenecteplase to first balloon inflation was 104 min. We noted the primary endpoint in 19% (151 of 810) of patients assigned facilitated PCI versus 13% (110 of 819) of those randomised to primary PCI (relative risk 1.39, 95% CI 1.11-1.74; p=0.0045). During hospital stay, significantly more strokes (1.8% [15 of 829] vs 0, p<0.0001), but not major non-cerebral bleeding complications (6% [46 of 829] vs 4% [37 of 838], p=0.3118), were reported in patients assigned facilitated rather than standard PCI. We also noted more ischaemic cardiac complications, such as reinfarction (6% [49 of 805] vs 4% [30 of 820], p=0.0279) or repeat target vessel revascularisation (7% [53 of 805] vs 3% [28 of 818], p=0.0041) within 90 days in this study group.

INTERPRETATION: A strategy of full-dose tenecteplase with antithrombotic co-therapy, as used in this study and preceding PCI by 1-3 h, was associated with more major adverse events than PCI alone in STEMI and cannot be recommended.

CARESS-IN-AMI

IMMEDIATE ANGIOPLASTY VERSUS STANDARD THERAPY WITH RESCUE ANGIOPLASTY AFTER THROMBOLYSIS IN THE COMBINED ABCIXIMAB RETEPLASE STENT STUDY IN ACUTE MYOCARDIAL INFARCTION (CARESS-IN-AMI): AN OPEN, PROSPECTIVE, RANDOMISED, MULTICENTRE TRIAL. LANCET. 2008.

This trial was done to study what is the optimal management of High risk ACS after thrombolysis at a non-interventional centre. Results showed that immediate transfer for PCI improves outcome in high-risk patients with STEMI treated at a non-interventional centre with half-dose reteplase and abciximab when compared with management in the local hospital with transfer only in case of persistent ST-segment

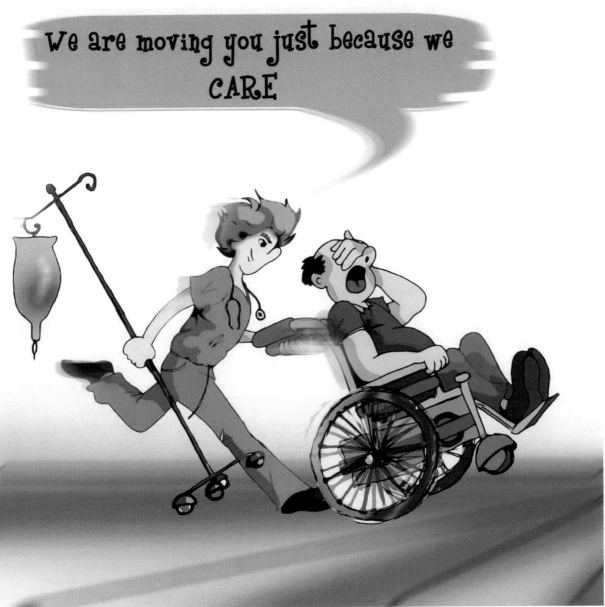

TRANSFER-AMI
ROUTINE EARLY ANGIOPLASTY AFTER FIBRINOLYSIS FOR ACUTE MYOCARDIAL INFARCTION.
NEW ENGLAND JOURNAL OF MEDICINE (NEJM) 2009.

This trial was done to study what is the optimal management of high risk ACS after thrombolysis at a non-interventional centre. Results showed that Among high-risk patients who had a myocardial infarction with ST-segment elevation and who were treated with fibrinolysis, transfer for PCI within 6 hours after fibrinolysis was associated with significantly fewer ischemic complications than was standard treatment.

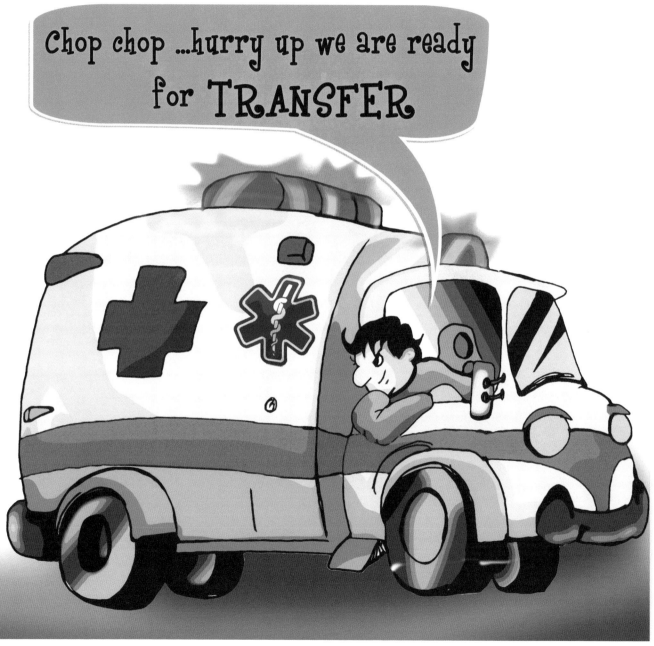

CARESS-In-AMI

Immediate angioplasty versus standard therapy with rescue angioplasty after thrombolysis in the Combined Abciximab REteplase Stent Study in Acute Myocardial Infarction (CARESS-in-AMI): an open, prospective, randomised, multicentre trial.

Di Mario C et al. CARESS-in-AMI (Combined Abciximab RE-teplase Stent Study in Acute Myocardial Infarction) Investigators.

Lancet. 2008; February16;371(9612):559-68.

BACKGROUND:
Thrombolysis remains the treatment of choice in ST-segment elevation myocardial infarction (STEMI) when primary percutaneous coronary intervention (PCI) cannot be done within 90 min. However, the best subsequent management of patients after thrombolytic therapy remains unclear. To assess the best management, we randomised patients with STEMI treated by thrombolysis and abciximab at a non-interventional hospital to immediate transfer for PCI, or to standard medical therapy with transfer for rescue angioplasty.

METHODS:
600 patients aged 75 years or younger with one or more high-risk features (extensive ST-segment elevation, new-onset left bundle branch block, previous myocardial infarction, Killip class >2, or left ventricular ejection fraction < or =35%) in hospitals in France, Italy, and Poland were treated with half-dose reteplase, abciximab, heparin, and aspirin, and randomly assigned to immediate transfer to the nearest interventional centre for PCI, or to management in the local hospital with transfer only in case of persistent ST-segment elevation or clinical deterioration. The primary outcome was a composite of death, reinfarction, or refractory ischaemia at 30 days, and analysis was by intention to treat. This study is registered with ClinicalTrials.gov, number 00220571.

FINDINGS: Of the 299 patients assigned to immediate PCI, 289 (97.0%) underwent angiography, and 255 (85.6%) received PCI. Rescue PCI was done in 91 patients (30.3%) in the standard care/rescue PCI group. The primary outcome occurred in 13 patients (4.4%) in the immediate PCI group compared with 32 (10.7%) in the standard care/rescue PCI group (hazard ratio 0.40; 95% CI 0.21-0.76, log rank p=0.004). Major bleeding was seen in ten patients in the immediate group and seven in the standard care/rescue group (3.4%vs 2.3%, p=0.47). Strokes occurred in two patients in the immediate group and four in the standard care/rescue group (0.7%vs 1.3%, p=0.50).

INTERPRETATION: Immediate transfer for PCI improves outcome in high-risk patients with STEMI treated at a non-interventional centre with half-dose reteplase and abciximab.

TRANSFER-AMI

Routine early angioplasty after fibrinolysis for acute myocardial infarction.

Cantor WJ et al.

New England Journal of Medicine (NEJM) 2009; June 25; 360(26):2705-18

BACKGROUND:

Patients with a myocardial infarction with ST-segment elevation who present to hospitals that do not have the capability of performing percutaneous coronary intervention (PCI) often cannot undergo timely primary PCI and therefore receive fibrinolysis. The role and optimal timing of routine PCI after fibrinolysis have not been established.

METHODS:

We randomly assigned 1059 high-risk patients who had a myocardial infarction with ST-segment elevation and who were receiving fibrinolytic therapy at centers that did not have the capability of performing PCI to either standard treatment (including rescue PCI, if required, or delayed angiography) or a strategy of immediate transfer to another hospital and PCI within 6 hours after fibrinolysis. All patients received aspirin, tenecteplase, and heparin or enoxaparin; concomitant clopidogrel was recommended. The primary end point was the composite of death, reinfarction, recurrent ischemia, new or worsening congestive heart failure, or cardiogenic shock within 30 days.

RESULTS:

Cardiac catheterization was performed in 88.7% of the patients assigned to standard treatment a median of 32.5 hours afterrandomization and in 98.5% of the patients assigned to routine early PCI a median of 2.8 hours after randomization. At 30 days, the primary end point occurred in 11.0% of the patients who were assigned to routine early PCI and in 17.2% of the patients assigned to standard treatment (relative risk with early PCI, 0.64; 95% confidence interval, 0.47 to 0.87; P=0.004). There were no significant differences between the groups in the incidence of major bleeding.

CONCLUSIONS:

Among high-risk patients who had a myocardial infarction with ST-segment elevation and who were treated with fibrinolysis, transfer for PCI within 6 hours after fibrinolysis was associated with significantly fewer ischemic complications than was standard treatment

OAT TRIAL

CORONARY INTERVENTION FOR PERSISTENT OCCLUSION AFTER MYOCARDIAL INFARCTION.
NEW ENGLAND JOURNAL OF MEDICINE (NEJM) 2006.

OAT trial tested the benefit of performing PCI on patients with acute MI and persistent occluded artery after a lag period of 3-28 days of the occurrence of the myocardial infarct. The results showed that PCI did not seem to help to reduce the rate of death, reinfarction, or heart failure in those patient compared to optimal medical therapy alone . On the contrary there was a trend toward excess reinfarction during the 4 years of follow-up.

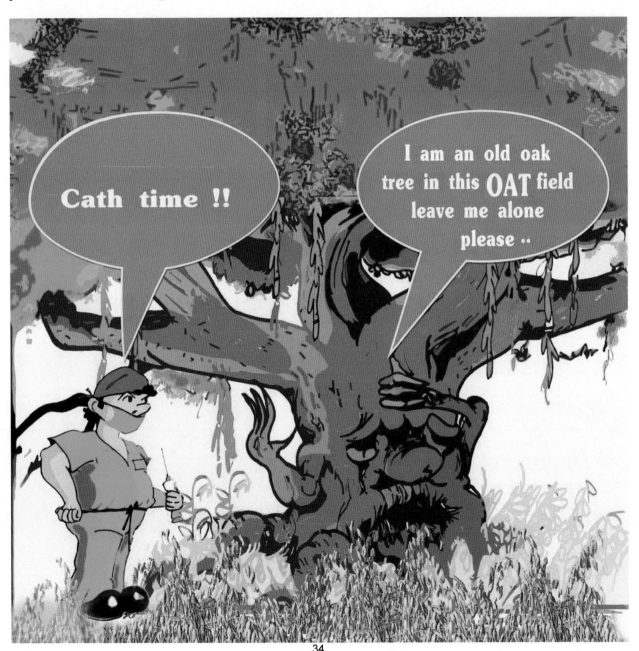

OAT Trial

Coronary intervention for persistent occlusion after myocardial infarction.

Hochman JS et al.

New England Journal of Medicine (NEJM) 2006; December 7; 355(23):2395-407.

BACKGROUND

It is unclear whether stable, high-risk patients with persistent total occlusion of the infarct-related coronary artery identified after the currently accepted period for myocardial salvage has passed should undergo percutaneous coronary intervention (PCI) in addition to receiving optimal medical therapy to reduce the risk of subsequent events.

METHODS

We conducted a randomized study involving 2166 stable patients who had total occlusion of the infarct-related artery 3 to 28 days aftermyocardial infarction and who met a high-risk criterion (an ejection fraction of <50% or proximal occlusion). Of these patients, 1082 were assigned to routine PCI and stenting with optimal medical therapy, and 1084 were assigned to optimal medical therapy alone. The primary end point was a composite of death, myocardial reinfarction, or New York Heart Association (NYHA) class IV heart failure.

RESULTS

The 4-year cumulative primary event rate was 17.2% in the PCI group and 15.6% in the medical therapy group (hazard ratio for death, reinfarction, or heart failure in the PCI group as compared with the medical therapy group, 1.16; 95% confidence interval [CI], 0.92 to 1.45; P=0.20). Rates of myocardial reinfarction (fatal and nonfatal) were 7.0% and 5.3% in the two groups, respectively (hazard ratio, 1.36; 95% CI, 0.92 to 2.00; P=0.13). Rates of nonfatal reinfarction were 6.9% and 5.0%, respectively (hazard ratio, 1.44; 95% CI, 0.96 to 2.16; P=0.08); only six reinfarctions (0.6%) were related to assigned PCI procedures. Rates of NYHA class IV heart failure (4.4% vs. 4.5%) and death (9.1% vs. 9.4%) were similar. There was no interaction between treatment effect and any subgroup variable (age, sex, race or ethnic group, infarct-related artery, ejection fraction, diabetes, Killip class, and the time from myocardial infarction to randomization).

CONCLUSIONS

PCI did not reduce the occurrence of death, reinfarction, or heart failure, and there was a trend toward excess reinfarction during 4 years of follow-up in stable patients with occlusion of the infarct-related artery 3 to 28 days after myocardial infarction.

Both these trials were done to look at thrombus aspiration in patients with STEMI, prior to primary percutaneous coronary intervention (PPCI) . The DEAR-MI study was a small study demonstrated that manual thrombus-aspirating before primary PCI, improved myocardial reperfusion compared with standard PPCI in patients with ST-segment elevation MI. TAPAS trial was a larger scale trial and confirmed that Thrombus aspiration results in better reperfusion and clinical outcomes than conventional PCI, irrespective of clinical and angiographic characteristics at baseline.

TAP..TAP.. my Deer

TAPA and DEAR-MI

DEAR-MI TRIAL

Thrombus aspiration before primary angioplasty improves myocardial reperfusion in acute myocardial infarction: the DEAR-MI (Dethrombosis to Enhance Acute Reperfusion in Myocardial Infarction) study.

Silva-Orrego P et al.

Journal of the American College of Cardiology. 2006, October 17; 48(8):1552-9.

OBJECTIVES: This study sought to test the hypothesis that thrombus removal, with a new manual thrombus-aspirating device, before primary percutaneous coronary intervention (PPCI) may improve myocardial reperfusion compared with standard PPCI in patients with ST-segment elevation acute myocardial infarction (STEMI).

BACKGROUND

In STEMI patients, PPCI may cause thrombus dislodgment and impaired microcirculatory reperfusion. Controversial results have been reported with different systems of distal protection or thrombus removal.

METHODS: One-hundred forty-eight consecutive STEMI patients, admitted within 12 h of symptom onset and scheduled for PPCI, were randomly assigned to PPCI (group 1) or manual thrombus aspiration before standard PPCI (group 2). Patients with cardiogenic shock, previous infarction, or thrombolytic therapy were excluded. Primary end points were complete (>70%) ST-segment resolution (STR) and myocardial blush grade (MBG) 3.

RESULTS

Baseline clinical and angiographic characteristics were similar in the 2 groups. Comparing groups 1 and 2: complete STR 50% versus 68% (p < 0.05); MBG-3 44% versus 88% (p < 0.0001); coronary Thrombolysis In Myocardial Infarction (TIMI) flow grade 3 78% versus 89% (p = NS); corrected TIMI frame count 21.5 +/- 12 versus 17.3 +/- 6 (p < 0.01); no reflow 15% versus 3% (p < 0.05); angiographic embolization 19% versus 5% (p < 0.05); direct stenting 24% versus 70% (p < 0.0001); and peak creatine kinase-mass band fraction 910 +/- 128 mug/l versus 790 +/- 132 mug/l (p < 0001). In-hospital clinical events were similar in the 2 groups. After adjusting for confounding factors, multivariate analysis showed thrombus aspiration to be an independent predictor of complete STR and MBG-3.

CONCLUSIONS

Manual thrombus aspiration before PPCI leads to better myocardial reperfusion and is associated with lower creatine kinase mass band fraction release, lower risk of distal embolization, and no reflow compared with standard PPCI.

TAPAS Trial

Thrombus aspiration during primary percutaneous coronary intervention.

Svilaas T et al.

New England Journal of Medicine (NEJM). 2008; February 7; 358(6):557-67.

BACKGROUND

Primary percutaneous coronary intervention (PCI) is effective in opening the infarct-related artery in patients with myocardial infarction with ST-segment elevation. However, the embolization of atherothrombotic debris induces microvascular obstruction and diminishes myocardial reperfusion.

METHODS

We performed a randomized trial assessing whether manual aspiration was superior to conventional treatment during primary PCI. A total of 1071 patients were randomly assigned to the thrombus-aspiration group or the conventional-PCI group before undergoing coronary angiography. Aspiration was considered to be successful if there was histopathological evidence of atherothrombotic material. We assessed angiographic and electrocardiographic signs of myocardial reperfusion, as well as clinical outcome. The primary end point was a myocardial blush grade of 0 or 1 (defined as absent or minimal myocardial reperfusion, respectively).

RESULTS

A myocardial blush grade of 0 or 1 occurred in 17.1% of the patients in the thrombus-aspiration group and in 26.3% of those in the conventional-PCI group (P<0.001). Complete resolution of ST-segment elevation occurred in 56.6% and 44.2% of patients, respectively (P<0.001). The benefit did not show heterogeneity among the baseline levels of the prespecified covariates. At 30 days, the rate of death in patients with a myocardialblush grade of 0 or 1, 2, and 3 was 5.2%, 2.9%, and 1.0%, respectively (P=0.003), and the rate of adverse events was 14.1%, 8.8%, and 4.2%, respectively (P<0.001). Histopathological examination confirmed successful aspiration in 72.9% of patients.

CONCLUSIONS

Thrombus aspiration is applicable in a large majority of patients with myocardial infarction with ST-segment elevation, and it results in better reperfusion and clinical outcomes than conventional PCI, irrespective of clinical and angiographic characteristics at baseline.

FAME AND FAME-2 TRIALS

The clinical utility of the ratio of maximal blood flow in a stenotic artery to normal maximal flow which is known as (FFR), was tested in FAME, and FAME-II trials. In Fame trial patients with multi-vessels disease were assigned t o get drug-eluting stents based on angiographic appearance in one group vs. FFR-significant lesions in the second group. The FFR-guided approach showed a decrease in the rate of the composite end point of death, nonfatal myocardial infarction, and repeat revascularization at 1 year. In FAME-II trial patients with stable CAD but functionally significant stenoses detected by FFR, PCI plus medical therapy will minimize the future need for urgent revascularization compared to the medical therapy alone.

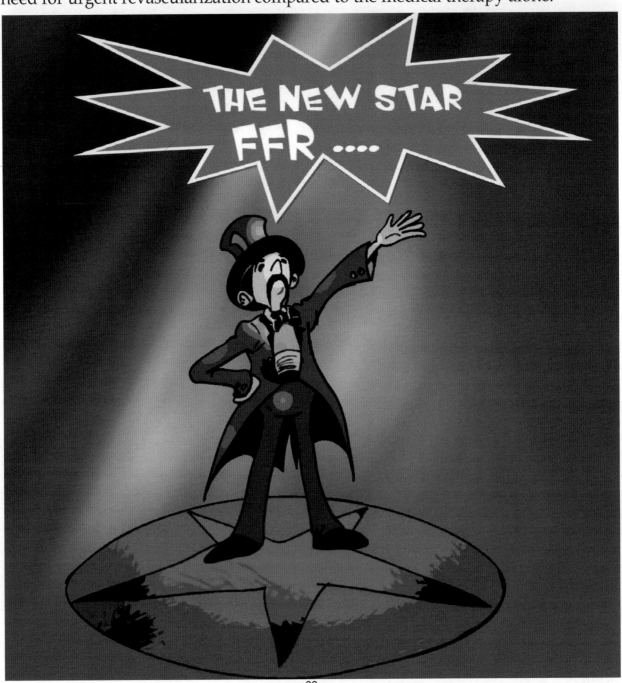

FAME TRIAL

Fractional flow reserve versus angiography for guiding percutaneous coronary intervention. Tonino PA et al.

New England Journal of Medicine (NEJM) 2009; January, 15;360(3):213-24.

BACKGROUND

In patients with multivessel coronary artery disease who are undergoing percutaneous coronary intervention (PCI), coronaryangiography is the standard method for guiding the placement of the stent. It is unclear whether routine measurement of fractional flow reserve (FFR; the ratio of maximal blood flow in a stenotic artery to normal maximal flow), in addition to angiography, improves outcomes.

METHODS

In 20 medical centers in the United States and Europe, we randomly assigned 1005 patients with multivessel coronary artery disease to undergo PCI with implantation of drug-eluting stents guided by angiography alone or guided by FFR measurements in addition to angiography. Before randomization, lesions requiring PCI were identified on the basis of their angiographic appearance. Patients assigned to angiography-guided PCI underwent stenting of all indicated lesions, whereas those assigned to FFR-guided PCI underwent stenting of indicated lesions only if the FFR was 0.80 or less. The primary end point was the rate of death, nonfatal myocardial infarction, and repeat revascularization at 1 year.

RESULTS

The mean (+/-SD) number of indicated lesions per patient was 2.7+/-0.9 in the angiography group and 2.8+/-1.0 in the FFR group (P=0.34). The number of stents used per patient was 2.7+/-1.2 and 1.9+/-1.3, respectively (P<0.001). The 1-year event rate was 18.3% (91 patients) in the angiography group and 13.2% (67 patients) in the FFR group (P=0.02). Seventy-eight percent of the patients in the angiography group were free from angina at 1 year, as compared with 81% of patients in the FFR group (P=0.20).

CONCLUSIONS

Routine measurement of FFR in patients with multivessel coronary artery disease who are undergoing PCI with drug-eluting stents significantly reduces the rate of the composite end point of death, nonfatal myocardial infarction, and repeat revascularization at 1 year.

FAME 2 Trial

Fractional flow reserve-guided PCI versus medical therapy in stable coronary disease. De Bruyne B et al. FAME 2 Trial Investigators.

New England Journal of Medicine (NEJM). 2012; September 13;367(11):991-1001

BACKGROUND

The preferred initial treatment for patients with stable coronary artery disease is the best available medical therapy. We hypothesized that in patients with functionally significant stenoses, as determined by measurement of fractional flow reserve (FFR), percutaneouscoronary intervention (PCI) plus the best available medical therapy would be superior to the best available medical therapy alone.

METHODS

In patients with stable coronary artery disease for whom PCI was being considered, we assessed all stenoses by measuring FFR. Patients in whom at least one stenosis was functionally significant (FFR, ≤0.80) were randomly assigned to FFR-guided PCI plus the best availablemedical therapy (PCI group) or the best available medical therapy alone (medical-therapy group). Patients in whom all stenoses had an FFR of more than 0.80 were entered into a registry and received the best available medical therapy. The primary end point was a composite of death, myocardial infarction, or urgent revascularization.

RESULTS

Recruitment was halted prematurely after enrollment of 1220 patients (888 who underwent randomization and 332 enrolled in the registry) because of a significant between-group difference in the percentage of patients who had a primary end-point event: 4.3% in the PCI group and 12.7% in the medical-therapy group (hazard ratio with PCI, 0.32; 95% confidence interval [CI], 0.19 to 0.53; P<0.001). The difference was driven by a lower rate of urgent revascularization in the PCI group than in the medical-therapy group (1.6% vs. 11.1%; hazard ratio, 0.13; 95% CI, 0.06 to 0.30; P<0.001); in particular, in the PCI group, fewer urgent revascularizations were triggered by a myocardial infarction or evidence of ischemia on electrocardiography (hazard ratio, 0.13; 95% CI, 0.04 to 0.43; P<0.001). Among patients in the registry, 3.0% had a primary end-point event.

CONCLUSIONS

In patients with stable coronary artery disease and functionally significant stenoses, FFR-guided PCI plus the best available medical therapy, as compared with the best available medical therapy alone, decreased the need for urgent revascularization. In patients without ischemia, the outcome appeared to be favorable with the best available medical therapy alone.

Unstable Angina/and Non-ST Segment Elevation Myocardial Infarction Trials

VA COOPERATIE AND RISC TRIALS

The VA COOPERATIE was the first to show the role that aspirin can play in the management of unstable angina. When compared with placebo, Aspirin showed a significant protective effect against acute myocardial infarction in men with unstable angina, without significant increase in the risk of GI Bleeding. In this study, however, there was no significant mortality benefit with aspirin. On the other hand RISC trial compared placebo with ASA alone, Heparin alone and ASA/Heparin. The study showed reduced event rate in non-Q-wave MI and unstable angina in the ASA and ASA/heparin group. Decreased mortality and MIs were noted in ASA and Heparin group during the first 5 days.

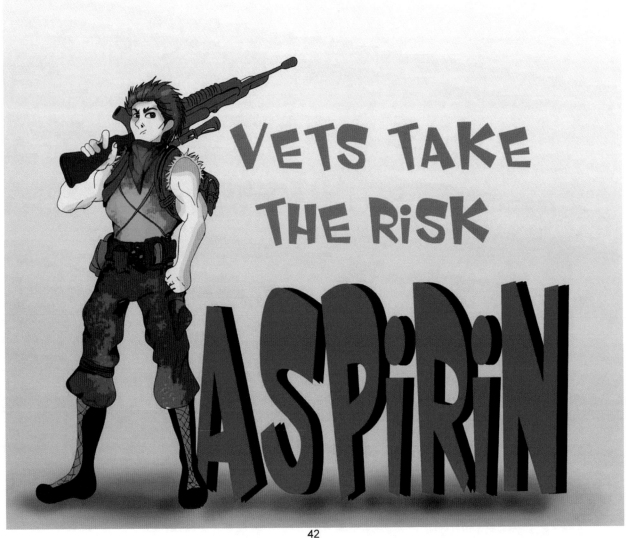

VETS TAKE THE RISK

ASPiRiN

VA COOPERATIE Trial: ASA

Protective effects of aspirin against acute myocardial infarction and death in men with unstable angina. Results of a Veterans Administration Cooperative Study.

Lewis HD Jr, et al.

New England Journal of Medicine (NEJM). 1983; August 18;309(7):396-403.

We conducted a multicenter, double-blind, placebo-controlled randomized trial of aspirin treatment (324 mg in buffered solution daily) for 12 weeks in 1266 men with unstable angina (625 taking aspirin and 641 placebo). The principal end points were death and acute myocardial infarction diagnosed by the presence of creatine kinase MB or pathologic Q-wave changes on electrocardiograms. The incidence of death or acute myocardial infarction was 51 per cent lower in the aspirin group than in the placebo group: 31 patients (5.0 per cent) as compared with 65 (10.1 per cent); P = 0.0005. Nonfatal acute myocardial infarction was 51 per cent lower in the aspirin group: 21 patients (3.4 per cent) as compared with 44 (6.9 per cent); P = 0.005. The reduction in mortality in the aspirin group was also 51 per cent--10 patients (1.6 per cent) as compared with 21 (3.3 per cent)--although it was not statistically significant; P = 0.054. There was no difference in gastrointestinal symptoms or evidence of blood loss between the treatment and control groups. Our data show that aspirin has a protective effect against acute myocardial infarction in men with unstable angina, and they suggest a similar effect on mortality.

RISC Trial

Risk of myocardial infarction and death during treatment with low dose aspirin and intravenous heparin in men with unstable coronary artery disease. The RISC Group.

Lancet. 1990 October 6;336(8719):827-30.796

Men with unstable coronary artery disease (unstable angina or non-Q-wave myocardial infarction [MI]), were randomised to double-blind placebo-controlled treatment with oral aspirin 75 mg/day and/or 5 days of intermittent intravenous heparin. The risk of MI and death was reduced by aspirin. After 5 days the risk ratio was 0.43 (confidence intervals, 0.21-0.91), at 1 month 0.31 (0.18-0.53), and at 3 months 0.36 (0.23-0.57). Aspirin reduced event rate in non-Q-wave MI and unstable angina, independently of electrocardiographic abnormalities or concurrent drug therapy. Heparin had no significant influence on event rate, although the group treated with aspirin and heparin had the lowest number of events during the initial 5 days. Treatment had few side-effects and high patient compliance.

CURE AND PCI-CURE TRIALS

CURE and PCI-CURE trials both established the role of Clopidogrel in patients with NSTEMI. In CURE trial long term use of clopidogrel in conjunction with aspirin decreased cardiovascular events, heart failure, revascularization and death, in patient presenting within 24 hours of NSTEMI. There was slight increase of non-life threatening bleeding. While in PCI-CURE trial compared pre-PCI dual antiplatelets treatment with clopidogrel followed by long-term therapy after PCI with a strategy of no pretreatment and short-term therapy for only 4 weeks after PCI. The early and long term use of dual anti-platelets was associated with decreased incidentce of a **composite** of cardiovascular death, MI, and revascularization. The results of this study **established the** common practice of "upstream" (prior to PCI) use of **clopidogrel**.

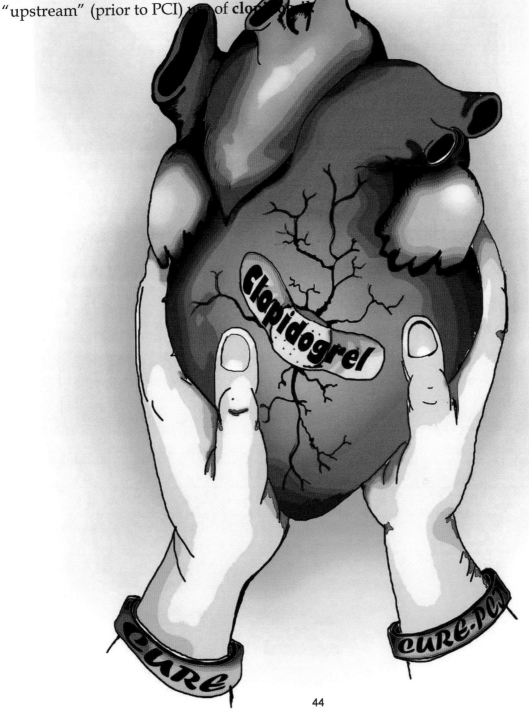

CURE TRIAL

Effects of clopidogrel in addition to aspirin in patients with acute coronary syndromes without ST-segment elevation.

Yusuf S, et al. Clopidogrel in Unstable Angina to Prevent Recurrent Events Trial Investigators.

New England Journal of Medicine (NEJM) 2001 August 16;345(7):494-502.

BACKGROUND: Despite current treatments, patients who have acute coronary syndromes without ST-segment elevation have high rates of major vascular events. We evaluated the efficacy and safety of the antiplatelet agent clopidogrel when given with aspirin in such patients.

METHODS: We randomly assigned 12,562 patients who had presented within 24 hours after the onset of symptoms to receive clopidogrel (300 mg immediately, followed by 75 mg once daily) (6259 patients) or placebo (6303 patients) in addition to aspirin for 3 to 12 months.

RESULTS: The first primary outcome--a composite of death from cardiovascular causes, nonfatal myocardial infarction, or stroke--occurred in 9.3 percent of the patients in the clopidogrel group and 11.4 percent of the patients in the placebo group (relative risk with clopidogrel as compared with placebo, 0.80; 95 percent confidence interval, 0.72 to 0.90; P<0.001). The second primary outcome--the first primary outcome or refractory ischemia--occurred in 16.5 percent of the patients in the clopidogrel group and 18.8 percent of the patients in the placebo group (relative risk, 0.86; 95 percent confidence interval, 0.79 to 0.94; P<0.001). The percentages of patients with in-hospital refractory or severe ischemia, heart failure, and revascularization procedures were also significantly lower with clopidogrel. There were significantly more patients with major bleeding in the clopidogrel group than in the placebo group (3.7 percent vs. 2.7 percent; relative risk, 1.38; P=0.001), but there were not significantly more patients with episodes of life-threatening bleeding (2.2 percent [corrected] vs. 1.8 percent; P=0.13) or hemorrhagic strokes (0.1 percent vs. 0.1 percent).

CONCLUSIONS: The antiplatelet agent clopidogrel has beneficial effects in patients with acute coronary syndromes without ST-segment elevation. However, the risk of major bleeding is increased among patients treated with clopidogrel.

PCI-CURE TRIAL

Effects of pretreatment with clopidogrel and aspirin followed by long-term therapy in patients undergoing percutaneous coronary intervention: the PCI-CURE study.

Mehta SR, et al. Clopidogrel in Unstable angina to prevent Recurrent Events trial (CURE) Investigators.

Lancet. 2001 August 18;358(9281):527-33.

BACKGROUND: Despite the use of aspirin, there is still a risk of ischaemic events after percutaneous coronary intervention (PCI). We aimed to find out whether, in addition to aspirin, pretreatment with clopidogrel followed by long-term therapy after PCI is superior to a strategy of no pretreatment and short-term therapy for only 4 weeks after PCI.

METHODS: 2658 patients with non-ST-elevation acute coronary syndrome undergoing PCI in the CURE study had been randomly assigned double-blind treatment with clopidogrel (n=1313) or placebo (n=1345). Patients were pretreated with aspirin and study drug for a median of 6 days before PCI during the initial hospital admission, and for a median of 10 days overall. After PCI, most patients (>80%) in both groups received open-label thienopyridine for about 4 weeks, after which study drug was restarted for a mean of 8 months. The primary endpoint was a composite of cardiovascular death, myocardial infarction, or urgent target-vessel revascularisation within 30 days of PCI. The main analysis was by intention to treat.

FINDINGS: There were no drop-outs. 59 (4.5%) patients in the clopidogrel group had the primary endpoint, compared with 86 (6.4%) in the placebo group (relative risk 0.70 [95% CI 0.50-0.97], p=0.03). Long-term administration of clopidogrel after PCI was associated with a lower rate of cardiovascular death, myocardial infarction, or any revascularisation (p=0.03), and of cardiovascular death or myocardial infarction (p=0.047). Overall (including events before and after PCI) there was a 31% reduction cardiovascular death or myocardial infarction (p=0.002). There was less use of glycoprotein IIb/IIIa inhibitor in the clopidogrel group (p=0.001). At follow-up, there was no significant difference in major bleeding between the groups (p=0.64).

INTERPRETATION: In patients with acute coronary syndrome receiving aspirin, a strategy of clopidogrel pretreatment followed by long-term therapy is beneficial in reducing major cardiovascular events, compared with placebo

TRITON-TIMI 38 AND TRILOGY-ACS TRIALS

TRITON-TIMI 38 showed that the Prasugrel (new thienopyridine) therapy in those undergoing PCI offered significant reduction in rates of ischemic events, including stent thrombosis, but with no mortality benefit and with an increased risk of major bleeding, including fatal bleeding. Subsequent TRILOGY ACS was done to see whether that benefit will sustain in those who are presenting with unstable angina or NSTEMI and are not planned to undergo PCI. Prasugrel was not associated with either a significant reduction in the frequency of the recurrent ischemic events or an increase risk of bleeding when compared with clopidogrel.

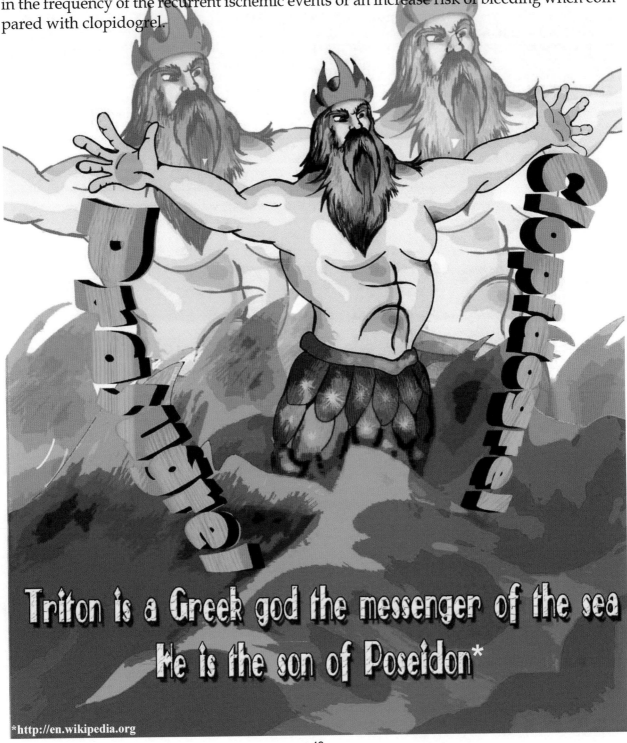

Triton is a Greek god the messenger of the sea
He is the son of Poseidon*

TRITON-TIMI 38 TRIAL

Prasugrel versus clopidogrel in patients with acute coronary syndromes.

Wiviott SD, et al. TRITON-TIMI 38 Investigators.

New England Journal of Medicine (NEJM) 2007; November 15; 357(20):2001-15.

BACKGROUND:

Dual-antiplatelet therapy with aspirin and a thienopyridine is a cornerstone of treatment to prevent thrombotic complications of acute coronary syndromes and percutaneous coronary intervention.

METHODS:

To compare prasugrel, a new thienopyridine, with clopidogrel, we randomly assigned 13,608 patients with moderate-to-high-risk acute coronary syndromes with scheduled percutaneous coronary intervention to receive prasugrel (a 60-mg loading dose and a 10-mg daily maintenance dose) or clopidogrel (a 300-mg loading dose and a 75-mg daily maintenance dose), for 6 to 15 months. The primary efficacy end point was death from cardiovascular causes, nonfatal myocardial infarction, or nonfatal stroke. The key safety end point was major bleeding.

RESULTS:

The primary efficacy end point occurred in 12.1% of patients receiving clopidogrel and 9.9% of patients receiving prasugrel (hazard ratio for prasugrel vs. clopidogrel, 0.81; 95% confidence interval [CI], 0.73 to 0.90; P<0.001). We also found significant reductions in the prasugrel group in the rates of myocardial infarction (9.7% for clopidogrel vs. 7.4% for prasugrel; P<0.001), urgent target-vessel revascularization (3.7% vs. 2.5%; P<0.001), and stent thrombosis (2.4% vs. 1.1%; P<0.001). Major bleeding was observed in 2.4% of patients receiving prasugrel and in 1.8% of patients receiving clopidogrel (hazard ratio, 1.32; 95% CI, 1.03 to 1.68; P=0.03). Also greater in the prasugrel group was the rate of life-threatening bleeding (1.4% vs. 0.9%; P=0.01), including nonfatal bleeding (1.1% vs. 0.9%; hazard ratio, 1.25; P=0.23) and fatal bleeding (0.4% vs. 0.1%; P=0.002).

CONCLUSIONS:

In patients with acute coronary syndromes with scheduled percutaneous coronary intervention, prasugrel therapy was associated with significantly reduced rates of ischemic events, including stent thrombosis, but with an increased risk of major bleeding, including fatal bleeding. Overall mortality did not differ significantly between treatment groups.

TRILOGY-ACS TRIAL.

Prasugrel versus clopidogrel for acute coronary syndromes without revascularization.

Roe MT, et al. TRILOGY ACS Investigators.

New England Journal of Medicine (NEJM) 2012; October 4;367(14):1297-309.

BACKGROUND:

The effect of intensified platelet inhibition for patients with unstable angina or myocardial infarction without ST-segment elevation who do not undergo revascularization has not been delineated.

METHODS:

In this double-blind, randomized trial, in a primary analysis involving 7243 patients under the age of 75 years receiving aspirin, we evaluated up to 30 months of treatment with prasugrel (10 mg daily) versus clopidogrel (75 mg daily). In a secondary analysis involving 2083 patients 75 years of age or older, we evaluated 5 mg of prasugrel versus 75 mg of clopidogrel.

RESULTS:

At a median follow-up of 17 months, the primary end point of death from cardiovascular causes, myocardial infarction, or stroke among patients under the age of 75 years occurred in 13.9% of the prasugrel group and 16.0% of the clopidogrel group (hazard ratio in the prasugrel group, 0.91; 95% confidence interval [CI], 0.79 to 1.05; P=0.21). Similar results were observed in the overall population. The prespecified analysis of multiple recurrent ischemic events (all components of the primary end point) suggested a lower risk for prasugrel among patients under the age of 75 years (hazard ratio, 0.85; 95% CI, 0.72 to 1.00; P=0.04). Rates of severe and intracranial bleeding were similar in the two groups in all age groups. There was no significant between-group difference in the frequency of nonhemorrhagic serious adverse events, except for a higher frequency of heart failure in the clopidogrel group.

CONCLUSIONS:

Among patients with unstable angina or myocardial infarction without ST-segment elevation, prasugrel did not significantly reduce the frequency of the primary end point, as compared with clopidogrel, and similar risks of bleeding were observed.

ESSENCE AND TIMI-11B TRIALS

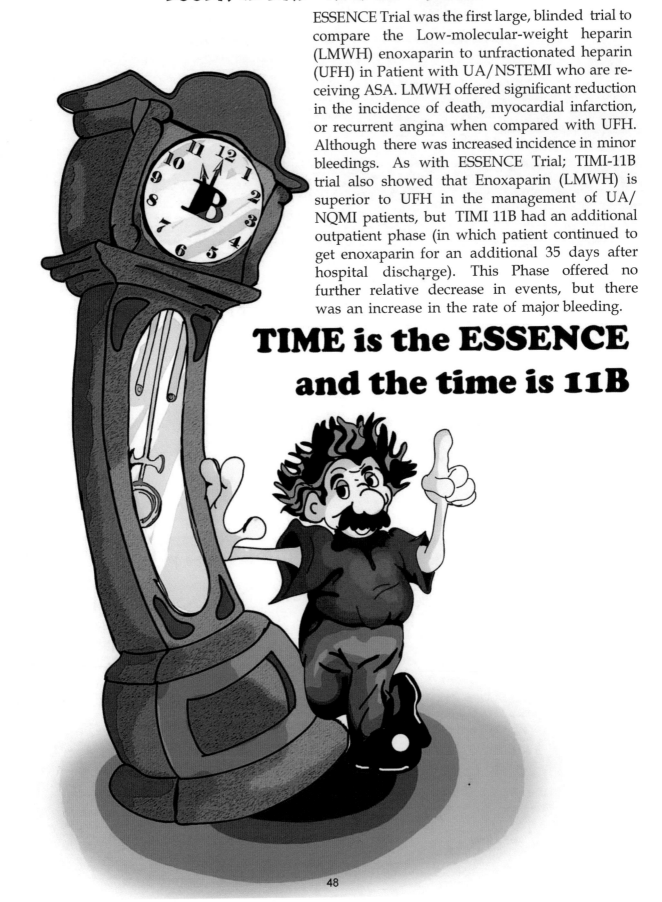

ESSENCE Trial was the first large, blinded trial to compare the Low-molecular-weight heparin (LMWH) enoxaparin to unfractionated heparin (UFH) in Patient with UA/NSTEMI who are receiving ASA. LMWH offered significant reduction in the incidence of death, myocardial infarction, or recurrent angina when compared with UFH. Although there was increased incidence in minor bleedings. As with ESSENCE Trial; TIMI-11B trial also showed that Enoxaparin (LMWH) is superior to UFH in the management of UA/NQMI patients, but TIMI 11B had an additional outpatient phase (in which patient continued to get enoxaparin for an additional 35 days after hospital discharge). This Phase offered no further relative decrease in events, but there was an increase in the rate of major bleeding.

TIME is the ESSENCE and the time is 11B

ESSENCE TRIAL

A comparison of low-molecular-weight heparin with unfractionated heparin for unstable coronary artery disease.
Efficacy and Safety of Subcutaneous Enoxaparin in Non-Q-Wave Coronary Events Study Group. Cohen M, et al.

New England Journal of Medicine (NEJM). 1997; August 14; 337(7):447-52.

BACKGROUND:

Antithrombotic therapy with heparin plus aspirin reduces the rate of ischemic events in patients with unstable coronary artery disease. Low-molecular-weight heparin has a more predictable anticoagulant effect than standard unfractionated heparin, is easier to administer, and does not require monitoring.

METHODS:

In a double-blind, placebo-controlled study, we randomly assigned 3171 patients with angina at rest or non-Q-wave myocardial infarction to receive either 1 mg of enoxaparin (low-molecular-weight heparin) per kilogram of body weight, administered subcutaneously twice daily, or continuous intravenous unfractionated heparin. Therapy was continued for a minimum of 48 hours to a maximum of 8 days, and we collected data on important coronary end points over a period of 30 days.

RESULTS:

At 14 days the risk of death, myocardial infarction, or recurrent angina was significantly lower in the patients assigned to enoxaparin than in those assigned to unfractionated heparin (16.6 percent vs. 19.8 percent, P=0.019). At 30 days, the risk of this composite end point remained significantly lower in the enoxaparin group (19.8 percent vs. 23.3 percent, P=0.016). The need for revascularization procedures at 30 days was also significantly less frequent in the patients assigned to enoxaparin (27.1 percent vs. 32.2 percent, P=0.001). The 30-day incidence of major bleeding complications was 6.5 percent in the enoxaparin group and 7.0 percent in the unfractionated-heparin group, but the incidence of bleeding overall was significantly higher in the enoxaparin group (18.4 percent vs. 14.2 percent, P=0.001), primarily because of ecchymoses at injection sites.

CONCLUSIONS:

Antithrombotic therapy with enoxaparin plus aspirin was more effective than unfractionated heparin plus aspirin in reducing the incidence of ischemic events in patients with unstable angina or non-Q-wave myocardial infarction in the early phase. This benefit of enoxaparin was achieved with an increase in minor but not in major bleeding.

TIMI-11B TRIAL

Enoxaparin prevents death and cardiac ischemic events in unstable angina/non-Q-wave myocardial infarction. Results of the thrombolysis in myocardial infarction (TIMI) 11B trial. Antman EM, et al.

Circulation. 1999 October 12;100(15):1593-601.

BACKGROUND:

Ticagrelor is an oral, reversible, direct-acting inhibitor of the adenosine diphosphate receptor P2Y12 that has a more rapid onset and more pronounced platelet inhibition than clopidogrel.

METHODS:

In this multicenter, double-blind, randomized trial, we compared ticagrelor (180-mg loading dose, 90 mg twice daily thereafter) and clopidogrel (300-to-600-mg loading dose, 75 mg daily thereafter) for the prevention of cardiovascular events in 18,624 patients admitted to the hospital with an acute coronary syndrome, with or without ST-segment elevation.

RESULTS:

At 12 months, the primary end point--a composite of death from vascular causes, myocardial infarction, or stroke--had occurred in 9.8% of patients receiving ticagrelor as compared with 11.7% of those receiving clopidogrel (hazard ratio, 0.84; 95% confidence interval [CI], 0.77 to 0.92; P<0.001). Predefined hierarchical testing of secondary end points showed significant differences in the rates of other composite end points, as well as myocardial infarction alone (5.8% in the ticagrelor group vs. 6.9% in the clopidogrel group, P=0.005) and death from vascular causes (4.0% vs. 5.1%, P=0.001) but not stroke alone (1.5% vs. 1.3%, P=0.22). The rate of death from any cause was also reduced with ticagrelor (4.5%, vs. 5.9% with clopidogrel; P<0.001). No significant difference in the rates of major bleeding was found between the ticagrelor and clopidogrel groups (11.6% and 11.2%, respectively; P=0.43), but ticagrelor was associated with a higher rate of major bleeding not related to coronary-artery bypass grafting (4.5% vs. 3.8%, P=0.03), including more instances of fatal intracranial bleeding and fewer of fatal bleeding of other types.

CONCLUSIONS:

In patients who have an acute coronary syndrome with or without ST-segment elevation, treatment with ticagrelor as compared with clopidogrel significantly reduced the rate of death from vascular causes, myocardial infarction, or stroke without an increase in the rate of overall major bleeding but with an increase in the rate of non-procedure-related bleeding.

SYNERGY TRIAL

ENOXAPARIN VS UNFRACTIONATED HEPARIN IN HIGH-RISK PATIENTS WITH NON-ST-SEGMENT ELEVATION ACUTE CORONARY SYNDROMES MANAGED WITH AN INTENDED EARLY INVASIVE STRATEGY: PRIMARY RESULTS OF THE SYNERGY RANDOMIZED TRIAL.
THE JOURNAL OF THE AMERICAN MEDICAL ASSOCIATION (JAMA). 2004; JULY 7.

This trial compared enoxaparin with unfractionated heparin (UFH) in high risk patients with non-ST-segment elevation ACS managed with an early invasive approach (Patient were higher risk patient for ischemic cardiac complications when compared to ESSENCE or TIMI-11B). Although Enoxaparin was not superior to UFH but it was non-inferior for the treatment of high-risk patients with NSTEMI. Enoxaparin use was associated modest increase of major bleeding.

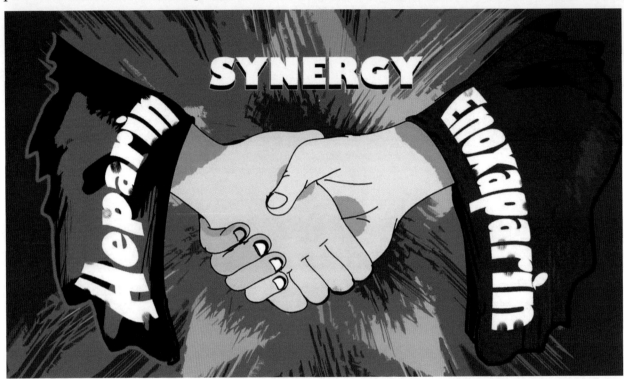

SYNERGY TRIAL

Enoxaparin vs unfractionated heparin in high-risk patients with non-ST-segment elevation acute coronary syndromes managed with an intended early invasive strategy: primary results of the SYNERGY randomized trial.
Ferguson JJ, et al.

The Journal of the American Medical Association (JAMA). 2004; July 7; 292(1):45-54.

CONTEXT:

Enoxaparin has demonstrated advantages over unfractionated heparin in low- to moderate-risk patients with non-ST-segment elevation acute coronary syndromes (ACS) treated with a conservative strategy.

OBJECTIVES:

To compare the outcomes of patients treated with enoxaparin vs unfractionated heparin and to define the role of enoxaparin in patients with non-ST-segment elevation ACS at high risk for ischemic cardiac complications managed with an early invasive approach.

DESIGN, SETTING, AND PARTICIPANTS:

The Superior Yield of the New Strategy of Enoxaparin, Revascularization and Glycoprotein IIb/IIIa Inhibitors (SYNERGY) trial was a prospective, randomized, open-label, multicenter, international trial conducted between August 2001 and December 2003. A total of 10 027 high-risk patients with non-ST-segment elevation ACS to be treated with an intended early invasive strategy were recruited.

INTERVENTIONS:

Subcutaneous enoxaparin (n = 4993) or intravenous unfractionated heparin (n = 4985) was to be administered immediately after enrollment and continued until the patient required no further anticoagulation, as judged by the treating physician.

MAIN OUTCOME MEASURES:

The primary efficacy outcome was the composite clinical end point of all-cause death or nonfatal myocardial infarction during the first 30 days after randomization. The primary safety outcome was major bleeding or stroke.

RESULTS:

The primary end point occurred in 14.0% (696/4993) of patients assigned to enoxaparin and 14.5% (722/4985) of patients assigned to unfractionated heparin (odds ratio [OR], 0.96; 95% confidence interval [CI], 0.86-1.06). No differences in ischemic events during percutaneous coronary intervention (PCI) were observed between enoxaparin and unfractionated heparin groups, respectively, including similar rates of abrupt closure (31/2321 [1.3%] vs 40/2364 [1.7%]), threatened abrupt closure (25/2321 [1.1%] vs 24/2363 [1.0%]), unsuccessful PCI (81/2281 [3.6%] vs 79/2328 [3.4%]), or emergency coronary artery bypass graft surgery (6/2323 [0.3%] vs 8/2363 [0.3%]). More bleeding was observed with enoxaparin, with a statistically significant increase in TIMI (Thrombolysis in Myocardial Infarction) major bleeding (9.1% vs 7.6%, P =.008) but nonsignificant excess in GUSTO (Global Utilization of Streptokinase and t-PA for Occluded Arteries) severe bleeding (2.7% vs 2.2%, P =.08) and transfusions (17.0% vs 16.0%, P =.16).

CONCLUSIONS:

Enoxaparin was not superior to unfractionated heparin but was noninferior for the treatment of high-risk patients with non-ST-segment elevation ACS. Enoxaparin is a safe and effective alternative to unfractionated heparin and the advantages of convenience should be balanced with the modest excess of major bleeding.

ACUITY TRIAL

BIVALIRUDIN FOR PATIENTS WITH ACUTE CORONARY SYNDROMES.

NEW ENGLAND JOURNAL OF MEDICINE (NEJM) 2006

ACUITY trial established the thrombin-specific anticoagulation with bivalirudin as a safe and effective alternative to UFH or the combination UFH/LMWH and GPIIb/IIIa inhibitors in patients with moderate- or high-risk acute coronary syndromes. Bivalirudin achieved the same reduction of rates of ischemia without an increased risk of bleeding when compared with heparin. As when compared to the combination of UFH and GPIIb/IIIa inhibitors; Bivalirudin alone achieved similar reduction of ischemia with significantly lower rates of bleeding.

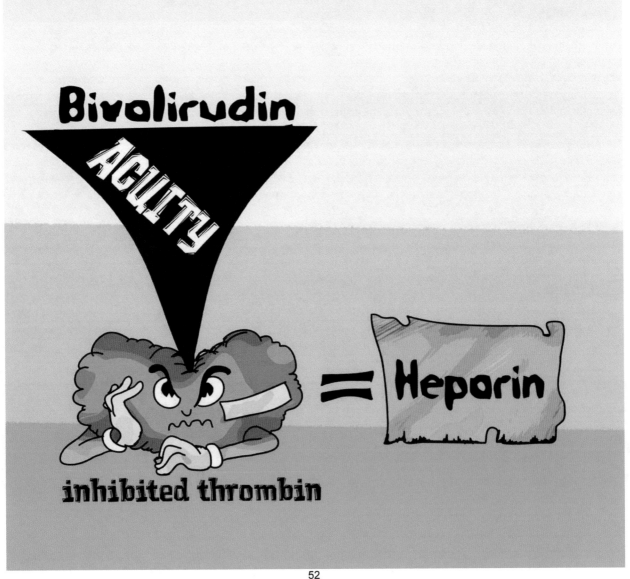

ACUITY TRIAL
Bivalirudin for patients with acute coronary syndromes.
Stone GW, et al.

New England Journal of Medicine (NEJM) 2006; November 23; 355(21):2203-16.

BACKGROUND:

Current guidelines for patients with moderate- or high-risk acute coronary syndromes recommend an early invasive approach with concomitant antithrombotic therapy, including aspirin, clopidogrel, unfractionated or low-molecular-weight heparin, and glycoprotein IIb/IIIa inhibitors. We evaluated the role of thrombin-specific anticoagulation with bivalirudin in such patients.

METHODS:

We assigned 13,819 patients with acute coronary syndromes to one of three antithrombotic regimens: unfractionated heparin or enoxaparin plus a glycoprotein IIb/IIIa inhibitor, bivalirudin plus a glycoprotein IIb/IIIa inhibitor, or bivalirudin alone. The primary end points were a composite ischemia end point (death, myocardial infarction, or unplanned revascularization for ischemia), major bleeding, and the net clinical outcome, defined as the combination of composite ischemia or major bleeding.

RESULTS:

Bivalirudin plus a glycoprotein IIb/IIIa inhibitor, as compared with heparin plus a glycoprotein IIb/IIIa inhibitor, was associated with noninferior 30-day rates of the composite ischemia end point (7.7% and 7.3%, respectively), major bleeding (5.3% and 5.7%), and the net clinical outcome end point (11.8% and 11.7%). Bivalirudin alone, as compared with heparin plus a glycoprotein IIb/IIIa inhibitor, was associated with a noninferior rate of the composite ischemia end point (7.8% and 7.3%, respectively; P=0.32; relative risk, 1.08; 95% confidence interval [CI], 0.93 to 1.24) and significantly reduced rates of major bleeding (3.0% vs. 5.7%; P<0.001; relative risk, 0.53; 95% CI, 0.43 to 0.65) and the net clinical outcome end point (10.1% vs. 11.7%; P=0.02; relative risk, 0.86; 95% CI, 0.77 to 0.97).

CONCLUSIONS:

In patients with moderate- or high-risk acute coronary syndromes who were undergoing invasive treatment with glycoprotein IIb/IIIa inhibitors, bivalirudin was associated with rates of ischemia and bleeding that were similar to those with heparin. Bivalirudin alone was associated with similar rates of ischemia and significantly lower rates of bleeding.

THE PRISM AND PRISM-PLUS TRIALS

Tirofiban is a GIIa/IIIb inhibitors that was studied in PRISM and PRISM-PLUS Trials. In PRISM trial tirofiban was compared to heparin. Patients with unstable angina, who did not go for revascularization, were randomized to receive 48 hours infusion of tirofiban versus heparin. Tirofiban showed benefits similar to heparin in decreasing events during the first 48 hours but not in 30 days. PRISM-PLUS trial had three arms comparing the tirofiban alone to heparin alone, and heparin plus tirofiban, in patients with unstable angina. Tirofiban alone showed increased short term mortality and that arm was prematurely terminated. While the combination of tirofiban plus heparin showed better outcome than heparin alone.

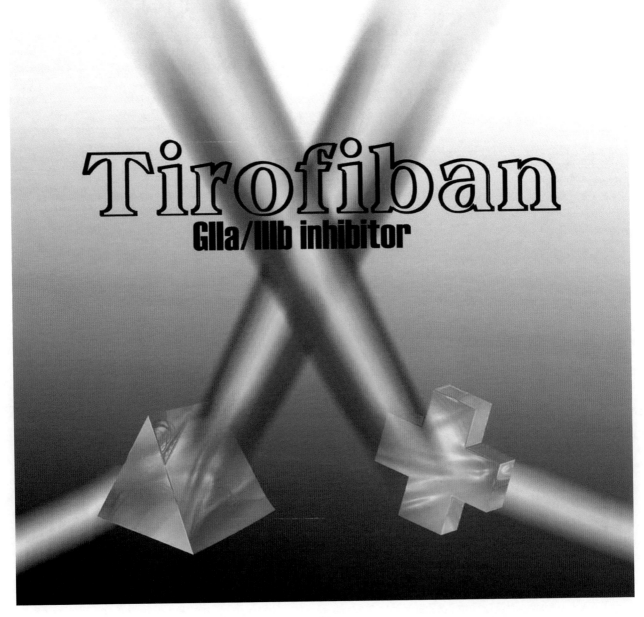

The PRISM TRIAL

A comparison of aspirin plus tirofiban with aspirin plus heparin for unstable angina. Platelet Receptor Inhibition in Ischemic Syndrome Management (PRISM) Study Investigators.

New England Journal of Medicine (NEJM). 1998; May 21; 338(21):1498-505.

BACKGROUND: Activation of platelets is central to the pathophysiology of unstable angina. We studied whether inhibition of the final common pathway for platelet aggregation with tirofiban, a nonpeptide glycoprotein IIb/IIIa receptor antagonist, would improve clinical outcome in this condition.

METHODS: In a double-blind study, we randomly assigned 3232 patients who were already receiving aspirin to additional treatment with intravenous tirofiban for 48 hours. The primary end point was a composite of death, myocardial infarction, or refractory ischemia at 48 hours.

RESULTS: The incidence of the composite end point was 32 percent lower at 48 hours in the group that received tirofiban (3.8 percent, vs. 5.6 percent with heparin; risk ratio, 0.67; 95 percent confidence interval, 0.48 to 0.92; P=0.01). Percutaneous revascularization was performed in 1.9 percent of the patients during the first 48 hours. At 30 days, the frequency of the composite end point (with the addition of readmission for unstable angina) was similar in the two groups (15.9 percent in the tirofiban group vs. 17.1 percent in the heparin group, P=0.34). There was a trend toward a reduction in the rate of death or myocardial infarction with tirofiban (a rate of 5.8 percent, as compared with 7.1 percent in the heparin group; risk ratio, 0.80; 95 percent confidence interval, 0.61 to 1.05; P=0.11), and mortality was 2.3 percent, as compared with 3.6 percent in the heparin group (P=0.02). Major bleeding occurred in 0.4 percent of the patients in both groups. Reversible thrombocytopenia occurred more frequently with tirofiban than with heparin (1.1 percent vs. 0.4 percent, P=0.04).

CONCLUSIONS: Tirofiban was generally well tolerated and, as compared with heparin, reduced ischemic events during the 48-hour infusion period, during which revascularization procedures were not performed. The incidence of refractory ischemia and myocardial infarction was not reduced at 30 days, but mortality was lower among the patients given tirofiban. Platelet inhibition with aspirin plus tirofiban may have a role in the management of unstable angina.

The PRISM PLUS TRIAL

Inhibition of the platelet glycoprotein IIb/IIIa receptor with tirofiban in unstable angina and non-Q-wave myocardial infarction. Platelet Receptor Inhibition in Ischemic Syndrome Management in Patients Limited by Unstable Signs and Symptoms (PRISM-PLUS) Study Investigators.

New England Journal of Medicine (NEJM). 1998; May 21; 338(21):1488-97.

BACKGROUND: Antithrombotic therapy improves the prognosis of patients with acute coronary syndromes, yet the syndromes remain a therapeutic challenge. We evaluated tirofiban, a specific inhibitor of the platelet glycoprotein IIb/IIIa receptor, in the treatment of unstable angina and non-Q-wave myocardial infarction.

METHODS: A total of 1915 patients were randomly assigned in a double-blind manner to receive tirofiban, heparin, or tirofiban plus heparin. Patients received aspirin if its use was not contraindicated. The study drugs were infused for a mean (+/-SD) of 71.3+/-20 hours, during which time coronary angiography and angioplasty were performed when indicated after 48 hours. The composite primary end point consisted of death, myocardial infarction, or refractory ischemia within seven days after randomization.

RESULTS: The study was stopped prematurely for the group receiving tirofiban alone because of excess mortality at seven days (4.6 percent, as compared with 1.1 percent for the patients treated with heparin alone. The frequency of the composite primary end point at seven days was lower among the patients who received tirofiban plus heparin than among those who received heparin alone (12.9 percent vs. 17.9 percent; risk ratio, 0.68; 95 percent confidence interval, 0.53 to 0.88; P=0.004). The rates of the composite end point in the tirofiban-plus-heparin group were also lower than those in the heparin-only group at 30 days (18.5 percent vs. 22.3 percent, P=0.03) and at 6 months (27.7 percent vs. 32.1 percent, P=0.02). At seven days, the frequency of death or myocardial infarction was 4.9 percent in the tirofiban-plus-heparin group, as compared with 8.3 percent in the heparin-only group (P=0.006). The comparable figures at 30 days were 8.7 percent and 11.9 percent (P=0.03), respectively, and those at 6 months were 12.3 percent and 15.3 percent (P=0.06). The benefit was consistent in the various subgroups of patients and in those treated medically as well as those treated with angioplasty. Major bleeding occurred in 3.0 percent of the patients receiving heparin alone and 4.0 percent of the patients receiving combination therapy (P=0.34).

CONCLUSIONS: When administered with heparin and aspirin, the platelet glycoprotein IIb/IIIa receptor inhibitor tirofiban was associated with a lower incidence of ischemic events in patients with acute coronary syndromes than in patients who received only heparin and aspirin.

EPIC and CAPTURE TRIALS

EPIC was the first trial to evaluate the role that platelet IIb/IIIa glycoprotein receptor inhibitors can play in high risk patients undergoing balloon angioplasty. Abciximab achieved significant reduction in the composite risk of death, MI , recurrent ischemia or failed angioplasty at 30 days. That was associated, however, with increased risk of bleeding. CAPTURE study established a short term (but not a long term) benefit of abciximab in patients with refractory unstable angina who are undergoing PTCA. Abciximab use was associated with significant reduction in the incidence of MI before, during PTCA. However, there was no long-term reduction in the rate of death, myocardial infarction or subsequent re-intervention.

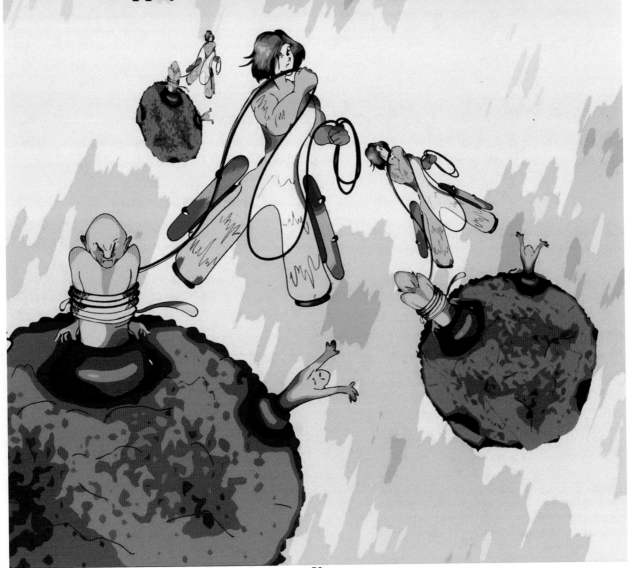

The EPIC of CAPTURING GP IIb/IIIa receptors

Abciximab is made from the Fab fragments of an immunoglobulin that targets the glycoprotein IIb/IIIa receptor on the platelet membrane

EPIC TRIAL.

Use of a monoclonal antibody directed against the platelet glycoprotein IIb/IIIa receptor in high-risk coronary angioplasty. The EPIC Investigation.
New England Journal of Medicine (NEJM). 1994; April 7; 330(14):956-61.

BACKGROUND:

Platelets are believed to play a part in the ischemic complications of coronary angioplasty, such as abrupt closure of the coronary vessel during or soon after the procedure. Accordingly, we evaluated the effect of a chimeric monoclonal-antibody Fab fragment (c7E3 Fab) directed against the platelet glycoprotein IIb/IIIa receptor, in patients undergoing angioplasty who were at high risk for ischemic complications. This receptor is the final common pathway for platelet aggregation.

METHODS:

In a prospective, randomized, double-blind trial, 2099 patients treated at 56 centers received a bolus and an infusion of placebo, a bolus of c7E3 Fab and an infusion of placebo, or a bolus and an infusion of c7E3 Fab. They were scheduled to undergo coronary angioplasty or atherectomy in high-risk clinical situations involving severe unstable angina, evolving acute myocardial infarction, or high-risk coronary morphologic characteristics. The primary study end point consisted of any of the following: death, nonfatal myocardial infarction, unplanned surgical revascularization, unplanned repeat percutaneous procedure, unplanned implantation of a coronary stent, or insertion of an intraaortic balloon pump for refractory ischemia. The numbers of end-point events were tabulated for 30 days after randomization.

RESULTS:

As compared with placebo, the c7E3 Fab bolus and infusion resulted in a 35 percent reduction in the rate of the primary end point (12.8 vs. 8.3 percent, P = 0.008), whereas a 10 percent reduction was observed with the c7E3 Fab bolus alone (12.8 vs. 11.5 percent, P = 0.43). The reduction in the number of events with the c7E3 Fab bolus and infusion was consistent across the end points of unplanned revascularization procedures and nonfatal myocardial infarction. Bleeding episodes and transfusions were more frequent in the group given the c7E3 Fab bolus and infusion than in the other two groups.

CONCLUSIONS:

Ischemic complications of coronary angioplasty and atherectomy were reduced with a monoclonal antibody directed against the platelet IIb/IIIa glycoprotein receptor, although the risk of bleeding was increased.

CAPTURE TRIAL

Randomised placebo-controlled trial of abciximab before and during coronary intervention in refractory unstable angina: the CAPTURE Study.
Lancet. 1997 May 17; 349(9063):1429-35.

BACKGROUND:

Platelet aggregation is a dominant feature in the pathophysiology of unstable angina. Percutaneous transluminal coronary angioplasty (PTCA) in patients with this disorder carries an increased risk of thrombotic complications. Abciximab (c7E3) blocks the platelet glycoprotein IIb/IIIa receptor, thus preventing platelet adhesion and aggregation. The CAPTURE study was a randomised placebo-controlled multicentre trial to assess whether abciximab can improve outcome in patients with refractory unstable angina who are undergoing PTCA.

METHODS:

The study recruited patients with refractory unstable angina, defined as recurrent myocardial ischaemia under medical treatment including heparin and nitrates. Predefined stopping rules were met at a planned interim analysis of data for 1050 patients, and recruitment was stopped. Data for 1265 patients (of 1400 scheduled) are presented here. After angiography, patients received a randomly assigned infusion of abciximab or placebo for 18-24 h before PTCA, continuing until 1 h afterwards. The primary endpoint was the occurrence within 30 days after PTCA of death (any cause), myocardial infarction, or urgent intervention for recurrent ischaemia. Analyses were by intention to treat.

FINDINGS:

By 30 days, the primary endpoint had occurred in 71 (11.3%) of 630 patients who received abciximab compared with 101 (15.9%) of 635 placebo recipients (p = 0.012). The rate of myocardial infarction was lower in the abciximab than in the placebo group before PTCA (four [0.6%] vs 13 [2.1%], p = 0.029) and during PTCA (16 [2.6%] vs 34 [5.5%], p = 0.009). Major bleeding was infrequent, but occurred more often with abciximab than with placebo (24 [3.8%] vs 12 [1.9%], p = 0.043). At 6-month follow-up, death, myocardial infarction, or repeat intervention had occurred in 193 patients in each group.

INTERPRETATION:

In patients with refractory unstable angina, treatment with abciximab substantially reduces the rate of thrombotic complications, in particular myocardial infarction, before, during, and after PTCA. There was no evidence that this regimen influenced the rate of myocardial infarction after the first few days, or the need for subsequent reintervention.

PURSUIT AND IMPACT-II TRIALS

Eptifibatide (Integrilin) is another GIIa/IIIb inhibitor that was evaluated in initially in two trials. PURSUIT trial showed that adding eptifibatide to heparin and aspirin in the setting of ACS (excluding STEMI) was associated with a reduction in mortality and MI. IMPACT-II looked at the effects of eptifibatide in patients with ACS undergoing PCI, it showed that infusion of Eptifibatide during coronary intervention reduced rates of early abrupt stent closure and ischemia.

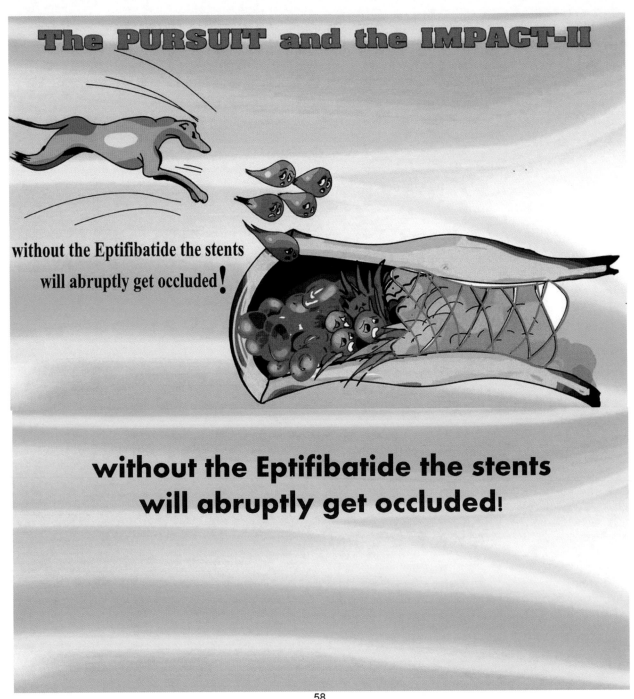

PURSUIT TRIAL

Inhibition of platelet glycoprotein IIb/IIIa with eptifibatide in patients with acute coronary syndromes. The PURSUIT Trial Investigators. Platelet Glycoprotein IIb/IIIa in Unstable Angina: Receptor Suppression Using Integrilin Therapy.

New England Journal of Medicine (NEJM) 1998; August; 13;339(7):436-43.

BACKGROUND:

Aggregation of platelets is the pathophysiologic basis of the acute coronary syndromes. Eptifibatide, a synthetic cyclic heptapeptide, is a selective high-affinity inhibitor of the platelet glycoprotein IIb/IIIa receptor, which is involved in platelet aggregation. We tested the hypothesis that inhibition of platelet aggregation with eptifibatide would have an incremental benefit beyond that of heparin and aspirin in reducing the frequency of adverse outcomes in patients with acute coronary syndromes who did not have persistent ST-segment elevation.

METHODS: Patients who had presented with ischemic chest pain within the previous 24 hours and who had either electrocardiographic changes indicative of ischemia (but not persistent ST-segment elevation) or high serum concentrations of creatine kinase MB isoenzymes were enrolled in the study. They were randomly assigned, in a double-blind manner, to receive a bolus and infusion of either eptifibatide or placebo, in addition to standard therapy, for up to 72 hours (or up to 96 hours, if coronary intervention was performed near the end of the 72-hour period). The primary end point was a composite of death and nonfatal myocardial infarction occurring up to 30 days after the index event.

RESULTS:

A total of 10,948 patients were enrolled between November 1995 and January 1997. As compared with the placebo group, the eptifibatide group had a 1.5 percent absolute reduction in the incidence of the primary end point (14.2 percent, vs. 15.7 percent in the placebo group; P=0.04). The benefit was apparent by 96 hours and persisted through 30 days. The effect was consistent in most major subgroups except for women (odds ratios for death or nonfatal myocardial infarction, 0.8 [95 percent confidence interval, 0.7 to 0.9] in men, and 1.1 [0.9 to 1.31 in women). Bleeding was more common in the eptifibatide group, although there was no increase in the incidence of hemorrhagic stroke.

CONCLUSIONS:

Inhibition of platelet aggregation with eptifibatide reduced the incidence of the composite end point of death or nonfatal myocardial infarction in patients with acute coronary syndromes who did not have persistent ST-segment elevation.

IMPACT-II TRIAL

Randomised placebo-controlled trial of effect of eptifibatide on complications of percutaneous coronary intervention: IMPACT-II. Integrilin to Minimise Platelet Aggregation and Coronary Thrombosis-II.

Lancet. 1997 May 17;349(9063):1422-8.

BACKGROUND:

Platelet-mediated thrombosis has been implicated in the development of ischaemic complications of percutaneous coronary intervention. We investigated whether inhibition of the platelet glycoprotein IIb/IIIa integrin with eptifibatide (Integrilin) could prevent such complications.

METHODS:

We undertook a double-blind, placebo-controlled trial at 82 centres in the USA, enrolling 4010 patients undergoing elective, urgent, or emergency coronary intervention. Patients were assigned one of three treatments: placebo (n = 1328), a bolus of 135 micrograms/kg eptifibatide followed by an infusion of 0.5 microgram kg-1 min-1 for 20-24 h (n = 1349), or 135 micrograms/kg eptifibatide bolus with a 0.75 microgram kg-1 min-1 infusion (n = 1333). The coronary procedure was started within 10-60 min of the start of study treatment. The primary endpoint was the 30-day composite occurrence of death, myocardial infarction, unplanned surgical or repeat percutaneous revascularisation, or coronary stent implantation for abrupt closure (by intention to treat). The primary safety endpoint was major bleeding.

FINDINGS:

By 30 days, the composite endpoint had occurred in 151 (11.4%) patients in the placebo group compared with 124 (9.2%) in the 135/0.5 eptifibatide group (p = 0.063) and 132 (9.9%) in the eptifibatide 135/0.75 group (p = 0.22). By treatment-received analysis, the 135/0.5 regimen produced a significant reduction in the composite endpoint (11.6 vs 9.1%, p = 0.035), but the 135/0.75 regimen produced a less substantial reduction (11.6 vs 10.0%, p = 0.18). Eptifibatide treatment did not increase rates of major bleeding or transfusion.

INTERPRETATION:

In the 135/0.5 group, treatment with eptifibatide during coronary intervention reduced rates of early abrupt closure and ischaemic events at 30 days. Non-significant differences were seen with the 135/0.75 regimen. The doses studied thus appear to be at the low end of the efficacy-response curve. Further investigation to refine eptifibatide dosing during coronary intervention is warranted.

FRISC-II, TACTICS, AND RITA-3 TRIALS

These three trials were one of the first to establish the role of early invasive strategy in management of patients with unstable angina conservative approach. FRISC-II study was the first trial to show the benefit of early invasive strategy in the management of NSTEMI, and the results were confirmed in TACTICS which showed that early use glycoprotein IIb/IIIa inhibitors in combination with an early invasive strategy, in intermediate and high risk patients, will significantly decrease the major cardiovascular events. RITA-3 on the other hand showed that early invasive strategy in low risk patients will improve angina symptoms although it didn't improve mortality in the low risk group.

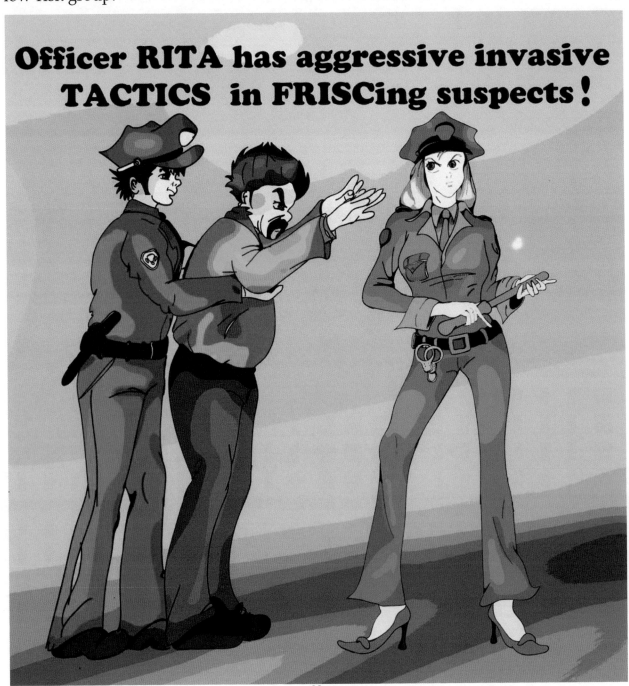

Officer RITA has aggressive invasive TACTICS in FRISCing suspects!

FRISC-II TRIAL
Invasive compared with non-invasive treatment in unstable coronary-artery disease: FRISC-II prospective randomised multicentre study. FRagmin and Fast Revascularisation during InStability in Coronary artery disease Investigators.
Lancet. 1999; August 28;354(9180):708-15.

BACKGROUND:

In unstable coronary-artery disease early invasive procedures are common, despite lack of evidence for the superiority of this approach. We compared an early invasive with a non-invasive treatment strategy in unstable coronary-artery disease.

METHODS:

In a prospective randomised multicentre study, we randomly assigned 2457 patients in 58 Scandinavian hospitals (median age 66 years, 70% men) an early invasive or non-invasive treatment strategy with placebo-controlled long-term low-molecular-mass heparin (dalteparin) for 3 months. Coronary angiography was done within the first 7 days in 96% and 10%, and revascularisation within the first 10 days in 71% and 9% of patients in the invasive and non-invasive groups, respectively. We followed up patients for 6 months. Analysis was by intention to treat.

FINDINGS:

After 6 months there was a decrease in the composite endpoint of death or myocardial infarction of 9.4% in the invasive group, compared with 12.1% in the non-invasive group (risk ratio 0.78 [95% CI 0.62-0.98], p=0.031). There was a significant decrease in myocardial infarction alone (7.8 vs 10.1%, 0.77 [0.60-0.99]; p=0.045) and non-significantly lower mortality (1.9 vs 2.9%, 0.65 [0.39-1.09]; p=0.10). Symptoms of angina and re-admission were halved by the invasive strategy. Results were independent of the randomised dalteparin treatment. The greatest advantages were seen in high-risk patients.

INTERPRETATION:

The early invasive approach should be the preferred strategy in most patients with unstable coronary-artery disease who have signs of ischaemia on electrocardiography or raised biochemical markers of myocardial damage

TACTICS-TIMI-18 TRIAL
Comparison of early invasive and conservative strategies in patients with unstable coronary syndromes treated with the glycoprotein IIb/IIIa inhibitor tirofiban.
Cannon CP, et al.
TACTICS (Treat Angina with Aggrastat and Determine Cost of Therapy with an Invasive or Conservative Strategy)--Thrombolysis in Myocardial Infarction 18 Investigators.
New England Journal of Medicine (NEJM) 2001; June 21; 344(25):1879-87.

BACKGROUND:

There is continued debate as to whether a routine, early invasive strategy is superior to a conservative strategy for the management of unstable angina and myocardial infarction without ST-segment elevation.

METHODS:

We enrolled 2220 patients with unstable angina and myocardial infarction without ST-segment elevation who had electrocardiographic evidence of changes in the ST segment or T wave, elevated levels of cardiac markers, a history of coronary artery disease, or all three findings. All patients were treated with aspirin, heparin, and the glycoprotein IIb/IIIa inhibitor tirofiban. They were randomly assigned to an early invasive strategy, which included routine catheterization within 4 to 48 hours and revascularization as appropriate, or to a more conservative (selectively invasive) strategy, in which catheterization was performed only if the patient had objective evidence of recurrent ischemia or an abnormal stress test. The primary end point was a composite of death, nonfatal myocardial infarction, and rehospitalization for an acute coronary syndrome at six months.

RESULTS:

At six months, the rate of the primary end point was 15.9 percent with use of the early invasive strategy and 19.4 percent with use of the conservative strategy (odds ratio, 0.78; 95 percent confidence interval, 0.62 to 0.97; P=0.025). The rate of death or nonfatal myocardial infarction at six months was similarly reduced (7.3 percent vs. 9.5 percent; odds ratio, 0.74; 95 percent confidence interval, 0.54 to 1.00; P<0.05).

CONCLUSIONS:

In patients with unstable angina and myocardial infarction without ST-segment elevation who were treated with the glycoprotein IIb/IIIa inhibitor tirofiban, the use of an early invasive strategy significantly reduced the incidence of major cardiac events. These data support a policy involving broader use of the early inhibition of glycoprotein IIb/IIIa in combination with an early invasive strategy in such patients.

RITA-3 TRIAL

Interventional versus conservative treatment for patients with unstable angina or non-ST-elevation myocardial infarction: the British Heart Foundation RITA 3 randomised trial. Randomized Intervention Trial of unstable Angina.

Fox KA, et al.

Lancet. 2002; September 7; 360(9335):743-51.

BACKGROUND:

Current guidelines suggest that, for patients at moderate risk of death from unstable coronary-artery disease, either an interventional strategy (angiography followed by revascularisation) or a conservative strategy (ischaemia-driven or symptom-driven angiography) is appropriate. We aimed to test the hypothesis that an interventional strategy is better than a conservative strategy in such patients.

METHODS:

We did a randomised multicentre trial of 1810 patients with non-ST-elevation acute coronary syndromes (mean age 62 years, 38% women). Patients were assigned an early intervention or conservative strategy. The antithrombin agent in both groups was enoxaparin. The co-primary endpoints were a combined rate of death, non-fatal myocardial infarction, or refractory angina at 4 months; and a combined rate of death or non-fatal myocardial infarction at 1 year. Analysis was by intention to treat.

FINDINGS:

At 4 months, 86 (9.6%) of 895 patients in the intervention group had died or had a myocardial infarction or refractory angina, compared with 133 (14.5%) of 915 patients in the conservative group (risk ratio 0.66, 95% CI 0.51-0.85, p=0.001). This difference was mainly due to a halving of refractory angina in the intervention group. Death or myocardial infarction was similar in both treatment groups at 1 year (68 [7.6%] vs 76 [8.3%], respectively; risk ratio 0.91, 95% CI 0.67-1.25, p=0.58). Symptoms of angina were improved and use of antianginal medications significantly reduced with the interventional strategy (p<0.0001).

INTERPRETATION:

In patients presenting with unstable coronary-artery disease, an interventional strategy is preferable to a conservative strategy, mainly because of the halving of refractory or severe angina, and with no increased risk of death or myocardial infarction.

TIMACS TRIAL

Early versus delayed invasive intervention in acute coronary syndromes.
Mehta SR, et al. TIMACS Investigators.

New England Journal of Medicine (NEJM) 2009 May 21;360(21):2165-75.

TIMACS trial was about the timing of the invasive strategy in patients with acute coronary syndromes, it hypothesized that earlier intervention (coronary angiography < or = 24 hours after randomization) could offer additional benefit over delayed intervention (coronary angiography > or = 36 hours after randomization). Results showed that although earlier intervention did not significantly reduce the primary outcome composite of death, myocardial infarction, or stroke at 6 months; it did significantly reduce the secondary composite of death, myocardial infarction, or refractory ischemia in high risk patients.

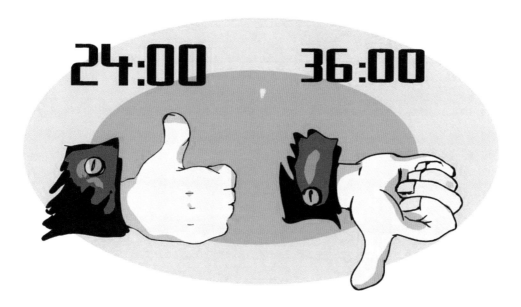

TIMACS Trial

BACKGROUND:
Earlier trials have shown that a routine invasive strategy improves outcomes in patients with acute coronary syndromes without ST-segment elevation. However, the optimal timing of such intervention remains uncertain.

METHODS:
We randomly assigned 3031 patients with acute coronary syndromes to undergo either routine early intervention (coronary angiography < or = 24 hours after randomization) or delayed intervention (coronary angiography > or = 36 hours after randomization). The primary outcome was a composite of death, myocardial infarction, or stroke at 6 months. A prespecified secondary outcome was death, myocardial infarction, or refractory ischemia at 6 months.

RESULTS: Coronary angiography was performed in 97.6% of patients in the early-intervention group (median time, 14 hours) and in 95.7% of patients in the delayed-intervention group (median time, 50 hours). At 6 months, the primary outcome occurred in 9.6% of patients in the early-intervention group, as compared with 11.3% in the delayed-intervention group (hazard ratio in the early-intervention group, 0.85; 95% confidence interval [CI], 0.68 to 1.06; P=0.15). There was a relative reduction of 28% in the secondary outcome of death, myocardial infarction, or refractory ischemia in the early-intervention group (9.5%), as compared with the delayed-intervention group (12.9%) (hazard ratio, 0.72; 95% CI, 0.58 to 0.89; P=0.003). Prespecified analyses showed that early intervention improved the primary outcome in the third of patients who were at highest risk (hazard ratio, 0.65; 95% CI, 0.48 to 0.89) but not in the two thirds at low-to-intermediate risk (hazard ratio, 1.12; 95% CI, 0.81 to 1.56; P=0.01 for heterogeneity).

CONCLUSIONS: Early intervention did not differ greatly from delayed intervention in preventing the primary outcome, but it did reduce the rate of the composite secondary outcome of death, myocardial infarction, or refractory ischemia and was superior to delayed intervention in high-risk patients.

MERLIN TIMI-36 TRIAL

EFFECTS OF RANOLAZINE ON RECURRENT CARDIOVASCULAR EVENTS IN PATIENTS WITH NON-ST-ELEVATION ACUTE CORONARY SYNDROMES: THE MERLIN-TIMI 36 RANDOMIZED TRIAL. JOURNAL OF THE AMERICAN MEDICAL ASSOCIATION (JAMA). 2007.

Ranolazine is believed to inhibit fatty acid oxidation, shift metabolism toward carbohydrate oxidation, and increase the efficiency of oxygen use. The MERLIN TIMI-36 trial enrolled patients with NSTEMI to be randomized to the addition of either Ranolazine or placebo to the standard medical therapy. There was no significant difference in the major cardiovascular events. However, there was a significant reduction in recurrent ischemia in the Ranolazine group. One of the other main findings of this trial was that the safety of ranolazine in terms of pro-arrhythmias as it is associated with prolonged QTc. As symptomatic documented arrhythmias did not differ between the two groups.

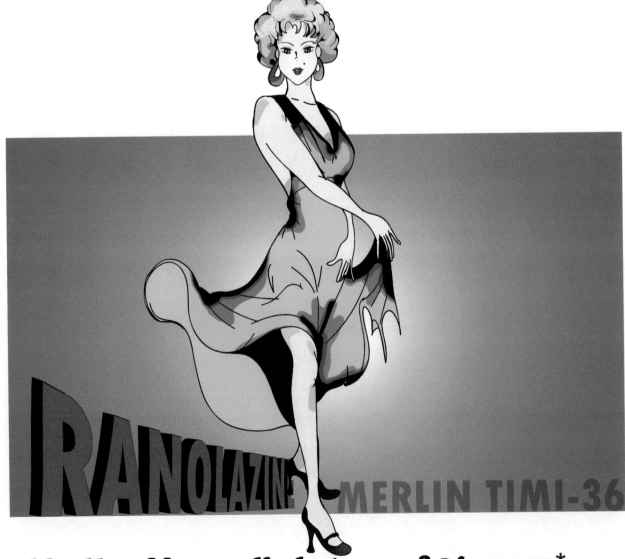

Marilyn Monro died at age of 36 years*

*http://en.wikipedia.org

MERLIN TIMI-36 trial

Effects of ranolazine on recurrent cardiovascular events in patients with non-ST-elevation acute coronary syndromes: the MERLIN-TIMI 36 randomized trial.

Morrow DA, et al.

Journal of the American Medical Association (JAMA). 2007; April 25; 297(16):1775-83.

CONTEXT:

Ranolazine is a novel antianginal agent that reduces ischemia in patients with chronic angina but has not been studied in patients with acute coronary syndromes (ACS).

OBJECTIVE:

To determine the efficacy and safety of ranolazine during long-term treatment of patients with non-ST-elevation ACS.

DESIGN, SETTING, AND PATIENTS:

A randomized, double-blind, placebo-controlled, multinational clinical trial of 6560 patients within 48 hours of ischemic symptoms who were treated with ranolazine (initiated intravenously and followed by oral ranolazine extended-release 1000 mg twice daily, n = 3279) or matching placebo (n = 3281), and followed up for a median of 348 days in the Metabolic Efficiency With Ranolazine for Less Ischemia in Non-ST-Elevation Acute Coronary Syndromes (MERLIN)-TIMI 36 trial between October 8, 2004, and February 14, 2007.

MAIN OUTCOME MEASURES:

The primary efficacy end point was a composite of cardiovascular death, myocardial infarction (MI), or recurrent ischemia through the end of study. The major safety end points were death from any cause and symptomatic documented arrhythmia.

RESULTS:

The primary end point occurred in 696 patients (21.8%) in the ranolazine group and 753 patients (23.5%) in the placebo group (hazard ratio [HR], 0.92; 95% confidence interval [CI], 0.83-1.02; P = .11). The major secondary end point (cardiovascular death, MI, or severe recurrent ischemia) occurred in 602 patients (18.7%) in the ranolazine group and 625 (19.2%) in the placebo group (HR, 0.96; 95% CI, 0.86-1.08; P = .50). Cardiovascular death or MI occurred in 338 patients (10.4%) allocated to ranolazine and 343 patients (10.5%) allocated to placebo (HR, 0.99; 95% CI, 0.85-1.15; P = .87). Recurrent ischemia was reduced in the ranolazine group (430 [13.9%]) compared with the placebo group (494 [16.1%]; HR, 0.87; 95% CI, 0.76-0.99; P = .03). QTc prolongation requiring a reduction in the dose of intravenous drug occurred in 31 patients (0.9%) receiving ranolazine compared with 10 patients (0.3%) receiving placebo. Symptomatic documented arrhythmias did not differ between the ranolazine (99 [3.0%]) and placebo (102 [3.1%]) groups (P = .84). No difference in total mortality was observed with ranolazine compared with placebo (172 vs 175; HR, 0.99; 95% CI, 0.80-1.22; P = .91).

CONCLUSIONS:

The addition of ranolazine to standard treatment for ACS was not effective in reducing major cardiovascular events. Ranolazine did not adversely affect the risk of all-cause death or symptomatic documented arrhythmia. Our findings provide support for the safety and efficacy of ranolazine as antianginal therapy

MIRACL AND PROVE IT TIMI-22 TRIALS

Before MIRACL trial, lipid-lower trials excluded patients with ACS, MIRACL Study came to establish the benefit of early initiation of statins therapy (atorvastatin 80 mg daily versus palcebo) in the management of ACS. While PROVE IT - TIMI22 was done to evaluate the best strategy in lowering LDL after ACS. PROVE IT - TIMI22 compared 40 mg of pravastatin daily (standard therapy) with 80 mg of atorvastatin daily (intensive therapy). It showed that more intensive strategy (with a goal of LDL <70) was associated with reduced death and major cardiovascular events.

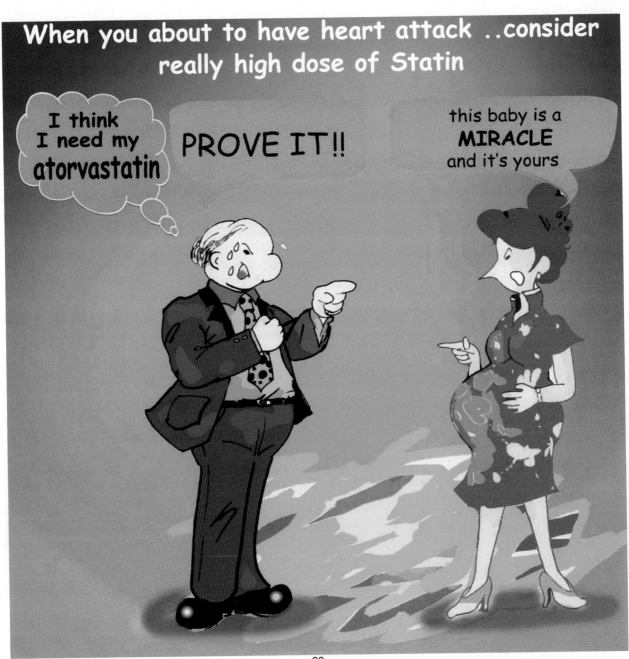

MIRACL TRIAL

Effects of atorvastatin on early recurrent ischemic events in acute coronary syndromes: the MIRACL study: a randomized controlled trial.

Schwartz GG, et al.

Journal of the American Medical Association (JAMA) 2001; April 4; 285(13):1711-8.

CONTEXT: Patients experience the highest rate of death and recurrent ischemic events during the early period after an acute coronary syndrome, but it is not known whether early initiation of treatment with a statin can reduce the occurrence of these early events.

OBJECTIVE: To determine whether treatment with atorvastatin, 80 mg/d, initiated 24 to 96 hours after an acute coronary syndrome, reduces death and nonfatal ischemic events.

DESIGN AND SETTING: A randomized, double-blind trial conducted from May 1997 to September 1999, with follow-up through 16 weeks at 122 clinical centers in Europe, North America, South Africa, and Australasia.

PATIENTS: A total of 3086 adults aged 18 years or older with unstable angina or non-Q-wave acute myocardial infarction.

INTERVENTIONS: Patients were stratified by center and randomly assigned to receive treatment with atorvastatin (80 mg/d) or matching placebo between 24 and 96 hours after hospital admission.

MAIN OUTCOME MEASURES: Primary end point event defined as death, nonfatal acute myocardial infarction, cardiac arrest with resuscitation, or recurrent symptomatic myocardial ischemia with objective evidence and requiring emergency rehospitalization.

RESULTS: A primary end point event occurred in 228 patients (14.8%) in the atorvastatin group and 269 patients (17.4%) in the placebo group (relative risk [RR], 0.84; 95% confidence interval [CI], 0.70-1.00; P =.048). There were no significant differences in risk of death, nonfatal myocardial infarction, or cardiac arrest between the atorvastatin group and the placebo group, although the atorvastatin group had a lower risk of symptomatic ischemia with objective evidence and requiring emergency rehospitalization (6.2% vs 8.4%; RR, 0.74; 95% CI, 0.57-0.95; P =.02). Likewise, there were no significant differences between the atorvastatin group and the placebo group in the incidence of secondary outcomes of coronary revascularization procedures, worsening heart failure, or worsening angina, although there were fewer strokes in the atorvastatin group than in the placebo group (12 vs 24 events; P =.045). In the atorvastatin group, mean low-density lipoprotein cholesterol level declined from 124 mg/dL (3.2 mmol/L) to 72 mg/dL (1.9 mmol/L). Abnormal liver transaminases (>3 times upper limit of normal) were more common in the atorvastatin group than in the placebo group (2.5% vs 0.6%; P<.001).

CONCLUSION: For patients with acute coronary syndrome, lipid-lowering therapy with atorvastatin, 80 mg/d, reduces recurrent ischemic events in the first 16 weeks, mostly recurrent symptomatic ischemia requiring rehospitalization.

PROVE IT - TIMI22 TRIAL

Intensive versus moderate lipid lowering with statins after acute coronary syndromes. Cannon CP, et al.

New England Journal of Medicine (NEJM). 2004; April 8; 350(15):1495-504.

BACKGROUND:

Lipid-lowering therapy with statins reduces the risk of cardiovascular events, but the optimal level of low-density lipoprotein (LDL) cholesterol is unclear.

METHODS:

We enrolled 4162 patients who had been hospitalized for an acute coronary syndrome within the preceding 10 days and compared 40 mg of pravastatin daily (standard therapy) with 80 mg of atorvastatin daily (intensive therapy). The primary end point was a composite of death from any cause, myocardial infarction, documented unstable angina requiring rehospitalization, revascularization (performed at least 30 days after randomization), and stroke. The study was designed to establish the noninferiority of pravastatin as compared with atorvastatin with respect to the time to an end-point event. Follow-up lasted 18 to 36 months (mean, 24).

RESULTS: The median LDL cholesterol level achieved during treatment was 95 mg per deciliter (2.46 mmol per liter) in the standard-dose pravastatin group and 62 mg per deciliter (1.60 mmol per liter) in the high-dose atorvastatin group (P<0.001). Kaplan-Meier estimates of the rates of the primary end point at two years were 26.3 percent in the pravastatin group and 22.4 percent in the atorvastatin group, reflecting a 16 percent reduction in the hazard ratio in favor of atorvastatin (P=0.005; 95 percent confidence interval, 5 to 26 percent). The study did not meet the prespecified criterion for equivalence but did identify the superiority of the more intensive regimen.

CONCLUSIONS:

Among patients who have recently had an acute coronary syndrome, an intensive lipid-lowering statin regimen provides greater protection against death or major cardiovascular events than does a standard regimen. These findings indicate that such patients benefit from early and continued lowering of LDL cholesterol to levels substantially below current target levels

Heart Failure Trials

DIG TRIAL

THE EFFECT OF DIGOXIN ON MORTALITY AND MORBIDITY IN PATIENTS WITH HEART FAILURE.
THE DIGITALIS INVESTIGATION GROUP.
NEW ENGLAND JOURNAL OF MEDICINE (NEJM) 1997.

DIG trial was the first trial that adequately powered to evaluate the effect of digoxin on mortality and hospitalization in patients with heart failure and normal sinus rhythm. It was done before the wide spread use of beta blockers for heart failure. Patients with a left ventricular ejection fraction of 0.45 or less were randomly assigned to digoxin or placebo. In this study digoxin did not reduce overall mortality or cardiovascular mortality, however it reduced overall hospitalizations and worsening of heart failure.

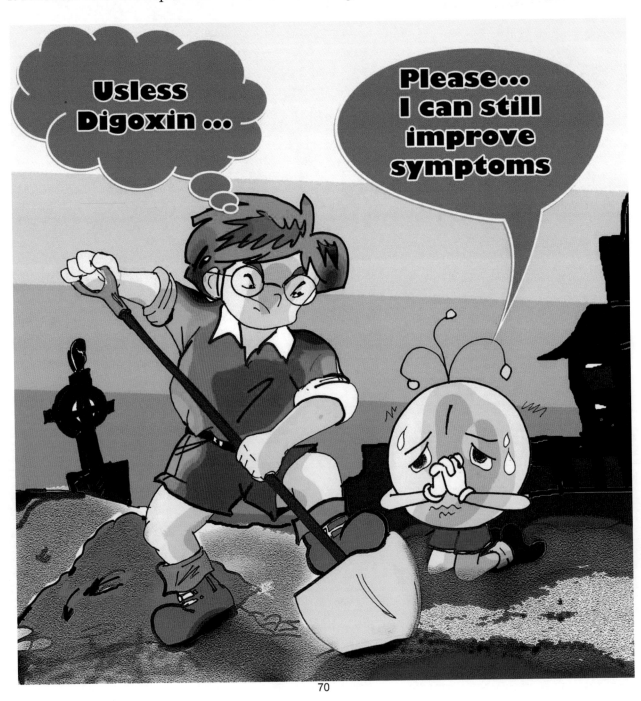

DIG TRIAL

The effect of digoxin on mortality and morbidity in patients with heart failure.

The digitalis investigation group.

New England Journal of Medicine (NEJM) 1997; February 20; 336(8):525-33

BACKGROUND:

The role of cardiac glycosides in treating patients with chronic heart failure and normal sinus rhythm remains controversial. We studied the effect of digoxin on mortality and hospitalization in a randomized, double-blind clinical trial.

METHODS:

In the main trial, patients with a left ventricular ejection fraction of 0.45 or less were randomly assigned to digoxin (3397 patients) or placebo (3403 patients) in addition to diuretics and angiotensin-converting-enzyme inhibitors (median dose of digoxin, 0.25 mg per day; average follow-up, 37 months). In an ancillary trial of patients with ejection fractions greater than 0.45, 492 patients were randomly assigned to digoxin and 496 to placebo.

RESULTS:

In the main trial, mortality was unaffected. There were 1181 deaths (34.8 percent) with digoxin and 1194 deaths (35.1 percent) with placebo (risk ratio when digoxin was compared with placebo, 0.99; 95 percent confidence interval, 0.91 to 1.07; $P=0.80$). In the digoxin group, there was a trend toward a decrease in the risk of death attributed to worsening heart failure (risk ratio, 0.88; 95 percent confidence interval, 0.77 to 1.01; $P=0.06$). There were 6 percent fewer hospitalizations overall in that group than in the placebo group, and fewer patients were hospitalized for worsening heart failure (26.8 percent vs. 34.7 percent; risk ratio, 0.72; 95 percent confidence interval, 0.66 to 0.79; $P<0.001$). In the ancillary trial, the findings regarding the primary combined outcome of death or hospitalization due to worsening heart failure were consistent with the results of the main trial.

CONCLUSIONS:

Digoxin did not reduce overall mortality, but it reduced the rate of hospitalization both overall and for worsening heart failure. These findings define more precisely the role of digoxin in the management of chronic heart failure

SOLVD TREATMENT AND SOLVD PREVENTION TRIALS

SOLVD trial was designed to study the effect of ACEI (enalapril) on mortality in patients with congestive heart failure (CHF). Patients with ejection fraction less than or equal to 0.35 were included in the (SOLVD treatment) trial if they had overt CHF and in the prevention trial if they were included in the prevention trial (SOLVD prevention). In the SOLV treatment trial patients were randomized to enalapril or placebo in addition to medical therapy (digitalis, diuretics, and vasodilators) and followed for over 41 months.

SOLVD treatment showed that enalapril therapy lowered mortality mainly by lowering mortality due to progressive heart failure in addition to lowering CHF hospitalizations. SOLVD prevention trial enrolled asymptomatic patients with known ejection fraction of 0.35 or less were not receiving therapy for heart failure. In SOLV prevention enalapril therapy significantly reduced the development and hospitalization for heart failure after an average follow up of over 37months. There was also a significant trend toward less cardiovascular mortality.

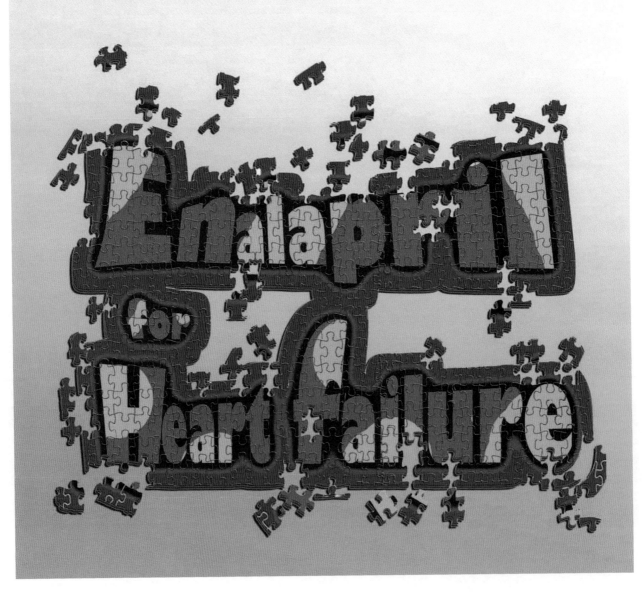

SOLVD TREATMENT TRIAL

Effect of enalapril on survival in patients with reduced left ventricular ejection fractions and congestive heart failure.

The SOLVD Investigators.

New England Journal of Medicine (NEJM). 1991; August 1; 325(5):293-302.

BACKGROUND:

Patients with congestive heart failure have a high mortality rate and are also hospitalized frequently. We studied the effect of an angiotensin-converting-enzyme inhibitor, enalapril, on mortality and hospitalization in patients with chronic heart failure and ejection fractions less than or equal to 0.35.

METHODS:

Patients receiving conventional treatment for heart failure were randomly assigned to receive either placebo (n = 1284) or enalapril (n = 1285) at doses of 2.5 to 20 mg per day in a double-bind trial. Approximately 90 percent of the patients were in New York Heart Association functional classes II and III. The follow-up averaged 41.4 months.

RESULTS:

There were 510 deaths in the placebo group (39.7 percent), as compared with 452 in the enalapril group (35.2 percent) (reduction in risk, 16 percent; 95 percent confidence interval, 5 to 26 percent; P = 0.0036). Although reductions in mortality were observed in several categories of cardiac deaths, the largest reduction occurred among the deaths attributed to progressive heart failure (251 in the placebo group vs. 209 in the enalapril group; reduction in risk, 22 percent; 95 percent confidence interval, 6 to 35 percent). There was little apparent effect of treatment on deaths classified as due to arrhythmia without pump failure. Fewer patients died or were hospitalized for worsening heart failure (736 in the placebo group and 613 in the enalapril group; risk reduction, 26 percent; 95 percent confidence interval, 18 to 34 percent; P less than 0.0001).

CONCLUSIONS:

The addition of enalapril to conventional therapy significantly reduced mortality and hospitalizations for heart failure in patients with chronic congestive heart failure and reduced ejection fractions.

SOLVD PREVENTION TRIAL

Effect of enalapril on mortality and the development of heart failure in asymptomatic patients with reduced left ventricular ejection fractions.

The SOLVD Investigators.

New England Journal of Medicine (NEJM) . 1992; December 10; 327(24):1768.

BACKGROUND:

It is not known whether the treatment of patients with asymptomatic left ventricular dysfunction reduces mortality and morbidity. We studied the effect of an angiotensin-converting--enzyme inhibitor, enalapril, on total mortality and mortality from cardiovascular causes, the development of heart failure, and hospitalization for heart failure among patients with ejection fractions of 0.35 or less who were not receiving drug treatment for heart failure.

METHODS:

Patients were randomly assigned to receive either placebo (n = 2117) or enalapril (n = 2111) at doses of 2.5 to 20 mg per day in a double-blind trial. Follow-up averaged 37.4 months.

RESULTS:

There were 334 deaths in the placebo group, as compared with 313 in the enalapril group (reduction in risk, 8 percent by the log-rank test; 95 percent confidence interval, -8 percent [an increase of 8 percent] to 21 percent; P = 0.30). The reduction in mortality from cardiovascular causes was larger but was not statistically significant (298 deaths in the placebo group vs. 265 in the enalapril group; risk reduction, 12 percent; 95 percent confidence interval, -3 to 26 percent; P = 0.12). When we combined patients in whom heart failure developed and those who died, the total number of deaths and cases of heart failure were lower in the enalapril group than in the placebo group (630 vs. 818; risk reduction, 29 percent; 95 percent confidence interval, 21 to 36 percent; P less than 0.001). In addition, fewer patients given enalapril died or were hospitalized for heart failure (434 in the enalapril group; vs. 518 in the placebo group; risk reduction, 20 percent; 95 percent confidence interval, 9 to 30 percent; P less than 0.001).

CONCLUSIONS:

The angiotensin-converting--enzyme inhibitor enalapril significantly reduced the incidence of heart failure and the rate of related hospitalizations, as compared with the rates in the group given placebo, among patients with asymptomatic left ventricular dysfunction. There was also a trend toward fewer deaths due to cardiovascular causes among the patients who received enalapril.

SAVE TRIAL

Effect of captopril on mortality and morbidity in patients with left ventricular dysfunction after myocardial infarction. Results of the survival and ventricular enlargement trial.

Pfeffer MA, et al. The SAVE Investigators.

New England Journal of Medicine (NEJM). 1992 September 3;327(10):669-77.

In patients who survived acute myocardial infarction, with asymptomatic LV dysfunction, captopril improved survival and decreased mortality and morbidity. The benefit was noted regardless of other medical therapies that the patients had received.

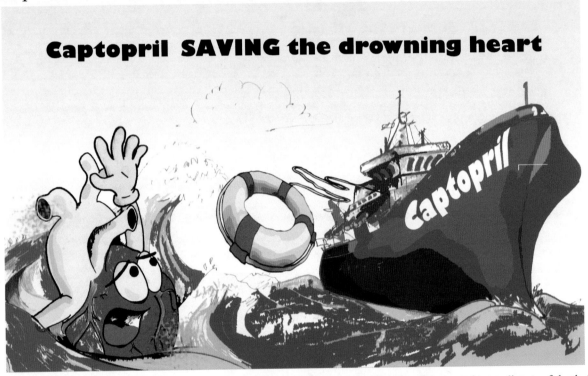

Captopril SAVING the drowning heart

BACKGROUND: Left ventricular dilatation and dysfunction after myocardial infarction are major predictors of death. In experimental and clinical studies, long term therapy with the angiotensin-converting--enzyme inhibitor captopril attenuated ventricular dilatation and remodeling. We investigated whether captopril could reduce morbidity and mortality in patients with left ventricular dysfunction after a myocardial infarction.

METHODS: Within 3 to 16 days after myocardial infarction, 2231 patients with ejection fractions of 40 percent or less but without overt heart failure or symptoms of myocardial ischemia were randomly assigned to receive doubleblind treatment with either placebo (1116 patients) or captopril (1115 patients) and were followed for an average of 42 months.

RESULTS: Mortality from all causes was significantly reduced in the captopril group (228 deaths, or 20 percent) as compared with the placebo group (275 deaths, or 25 percent); the reduction in risk was 19 percent (95 percent confidence interval, 3 to 32 percent; P = 0.019). In addition, the incidence of both fatal and nonfatal major cardiovascular events was consistently reduced in the captopril group. The reduction in risk was 21 percent (95 percent confidence interval, 5 to 35 percent; P = 0.014) for death from cardiovascular causes, 37 percent (95 percent confidence interval, 20 to 50 percent; P less than 0.001) for the development of severe heart failure, 22 percent (95 percent confidence interval, 4 to 37 percent; P = 0.019) for congestive heart failure requiring hospitalization, and 25 percent (95 percent confidence interval, 5 to 40 percent; P = 0.015) for recurrent myocardial infarction.

CONCLUSIONS: In patients with asymptomatic left ventricular dysfunction after myocardial infarction, long-term administration of captopril was associated with an improvement in survival and reduced morbidity and mortality due to major cardiovascular events. These benefits were observed in patients who received thrombolytic therapy, aspirin, or beta-blockers, as well as those who did not, suggesting that treatment with captopril leads to additional improvement in outcome among selected survivors of myocardial infarction.

ATLAS TRIAL
COMPARATIVE EFFECTS OF LOW AND HIGH DOSES OF THE ANGIOTENSIN-CONVERTING ENZYME INHIBITOR, LISINOPRIL, ON MORBIDITY AND MORTALITY IN CHRONIC HEART FAILURE. CIRCULATION. 1999.

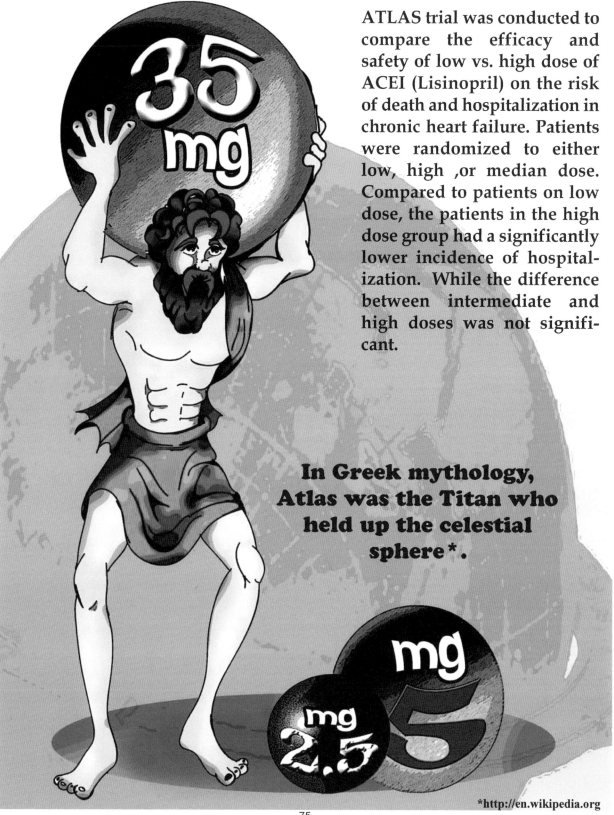

ATLAS trial was conducted to compare the efficacy and safety of low vs. high dose of ACEI (Lisinopril) on the risk of death and hospitalization in chronic heart failure. Patients were randomized to either low, high, or median dose. Compared to patients on low dose, the patients in the high dose group had a significantly lower incidence of hospitalization. While the difference between intermediate and high doses was not significant.

In Greek mythology, Atlas was the Titan who held up the celestial sphere*.

*http://en.wikipedia.org

ATLAS TRIAL
Comparative Effects of Low and High Doses of the Angiotensin-Converting Enzyme Inhibitor, Lisinopril, on Morbidity and Mortality in Chronic Heart Failure.
Packer M, et al.

Circulation. 1999; December 7; 100(23):2312-8

BACKGROUND:

Angiotensin-converting enzyme (ACE) inhibitors are generally prescribed by physicians in doses lower than the large doses that have been shown to reduce morbidity and mortality in patients with heart failure. It is unclear, however, if low doses and high doses of ACE inhibitors have similar benefits.

METHODS AND RESULTS:

We randomly assigned 3164 patients with New York Heart Association class II to IV heart failure and an ejection fraction < or = 30% to double-blind treatment with either low doses (2.5 to 5.0 mg daily, n=1596) or high doses (32.5 to 35 mg daily, n=1568) of the ACE inhibitor, lisinopril, for 39 to 58 months, while background therapy for heart failure was continued. When compared with the low-dose group, patients in the high-dose group had a non-significant 8% lower risk of death (P=0.128) but a significant 12% lower risk of death or hospitalization for any reason (P=0.002) and 24% fewer hospitalizations for heart failure (P=0.002). Dizziness and renal insufficiency was observed more frequently in the high-dose group, but the 2 groups were similar in the number of patients requiring discontinuation of the study medication.

CONCLUSION:

These findings indicate that patients with heart failure should not generally be maintained on very low doses of an ACE inhibitor (unless these are the only doses that can be tolerated) and suggest that the difference in efficacy between intermediate and high doses of an ACE inhibitor (if any) is likely to be very small.

CHARM TRIALS LANCET. 2003

CHARM-Preserved: included patients with LVEF higher than 40%.

CHARM trial was designed to investigate the effects of ARB on patients with CHF. Patients with heart failure (NYHA II-IV) were enrolled in one of three branches of the trial done in parallel manner to receive ARB (Candesartan) or placebo. In all the three trials candesartan lowered cardiovascular mortality as well as reduced hospital admissions for heart failure.

CHARM-Added: included patients with LVEF 40% or lower and being treated with ACEI.

CHARM-Alternative: included patients with LVEF 40% or lower intolerant to ACEI.

CANDESARTAN

CHARM overall

Effects of candesartan on mortality and morbidity in patients with chronic heart failure: the CHARM-Overall program.   Pfeffer MA, et al.

Lancet. 2003; September 6;362(9386):759-66.

BACKGROUND:

Patients with chronic heart failure (CHF) are at high risk of cardiovascular death and recurrent hospital admissions. We aimed to find out whether the use of an angiotensin-receptor blocker could reduce mortality and morbidity.

METHODS:

In parallel, randomized, double-blind, controlled, clinical trials we compared candesartan with placebo in three distinct populations. We studied patients with left-ventricular ejection fraction (LVEF) 40% or less who were not receiving angiotensin-converting-enzyme inhibitors because of previous intolerance or who were currently receiving angiotensin-converting-enzyme inhibitors, and patients with LVEF higher than 40%. Overall, 7601patients (7599 with data) were randomly assigned candesartan (n=3803, titrated to 32 mg once daily) or matching placebo (n=3796), and followed up for at least 2 years. The primary outcome of the overall programme was all-cause mortality, and for all the component trials was cardiovascular death or hospital admission for CHF. Analysis was by intention to treat.

FINDINGS:

Median follow-up was 37.7 months. 886 (23%) patients in the candesartan and 945 (25%) in the placebo group died (unadjusted hazard ratio 0.91 [95% CI 0.83-1.00], p=0.055; covariate adjusted 0.90 [0.82-0.99], p=0.032), with fewer cardiovascular deaths (691 [18%] vs 769 [20%], unadjusted 0.88 [0.79-0.97], p=0.012; covariate adjusted 0.87 [0.78-0.96], p=0.006) and hospital admissions for CHF (757 [20%] vs 918 [24%], p<0.0001) in the candesartan group. There was no significant heterogeneity for candesartan results across the component trials. More patients discontinued candesartan than placebo because of concerns about renal function, hypotension, and hyperkalaemia.

INTERPRETATION:

Candesartan was generally well tolerated and significantly reduced cardiovascular deaths and hospital admissions for heart failure. Ejection fraction or treatment at baseline did not alter these effects.

CHARM Preserved

Effects of candesartan in patients with chronic heart failure and preserved left-ventricular ejection fraction: the CHARM Preserved Trial.

Yusuf S, et al.

Lancet. 2003; September 6;362(9386):777-81.

BACKGROUND:

Half of patients with chronic heart failure (CHF) have preserved left-ventricular ejection fraction (LVEF), but few treatments have specifically been assessed in such patients. In previous studies of patients with CHF and low LVEF or vascular disease and preserved LVEF, inhibition of the renin-angiotensin system is beneficial. We investigated the effect of addition of an angiotensin-receptor blocker to current treatments.

METHODS:

Between March, 1999, and July, 2000, we randomly assigned 3023 patients candesartan (n=1514, target dose 32 mg once daily) or matching placebo (n=1509). Patients had New York Heart Association functional class II-IV CHF and LVEF higher than 40%. The primary outcome was cardiovascular death or admission to hospital for CHF. Analysis was done by intention to treat.

FINDINGS:

Median follow-up was 36.6 months. 333 (22%) patients in the candesartan and 366 (24%) in the placebo group experienced the primary outcome (unadjusted hazard ratio 0.89 [95% CI 0.77-1.03], p=0.118; covariate adjusted 0.86 [0.74-1.0], p=0.051). Cardiovascular death did not differ between groups (170 vs 170), but fewer patients in the candesartan group than in the placebo group were admitted to hospital for CHF once (230 vs 279, p=0.017) or multiple times. Composite outcomes that included non-fatal myocardial infarction and non-fatal stroke showed similar results to the primary composite (388 vs 429; unadjusted 0.88 [0.77-1.01], p=0.078; covariate adjusted 0.86 [0.75-0.99], p=0.037).

INTERPRETATION:

Candesartan has a moderate impact in preventing admissions for CHF among patients who have heart failure and LVEF higher than 40%.

CHARM Added

Effects of candesartan in patients with chronic heart failure and reduced left-ventricular systolic function taking angiotensinconverting-enzyme inhibitors: the CHARM-Added trial. McMurray JJ, et al.

Lancet. 2003 September 6;362(9386):767-71.

BACKGROUND:

Angiotensin II type 1 receptor blockers have favorable effects on hemodynamic measurements, neurohumoral activity, and left-ventricular remodeling when added to angiotensin-converting-enzyme (ACE) inhibitors in patients with chronic heart failure (CHF). We aimed to find out whether these drugs improve clinical outcome.

METHODS:

Between March, 1999, and November, 1999, we enrolled 2548 patients with New York Heart Association functional class II-IV CHF and left-ventricular ejection fraction 40% or lower, and who were being treated with ACE inhibitors. We randomly assigned patients candesartan (n=1276, target dose 32 mg once daily) or placebo (n=1272). At baseline, 55% of patients were also treated with beta blockers and 17% with spironolactone. The primary outcome of the study was the composite of cardiovascular death or hospital admission for CHF. Analysis was done by intention to treat.

FINDINGS:

The median follow-up was 41 months. 483 (38%) patients in the candesartan group and 538 (42%) in the placebo group experienced the primary outcome (unadjusted hazard ratio 0.85 [95% CI 0.75-0.96], p=0.011; covariate adjusted p=0.010). Candesartan reduced each of the components of the primary outcome significantly, as well as the total number of hospital admissions for CHF. The benefits of candesartan were similar in all predefined subgroups, including patients receiving baseline beta blocker treatment.

INTERPRETATION:

The addition of candesartan to ACE inhibitor and other treatment leads to a further clinically important reduction in relevant cardiovascular events in patients with CHF and reduced left-ventricular ejection fraction.

CHARM Alternative

Effects of candesartan in patients with chronic heart failureand reduced left-ventricular systolic function intolerant to angiotensin-converting-enzyme inhibitors: the CHARM-Alternative trial Granger CB, et al.

Lancet. 2003 September 6;362(9386):772-6.

BACKGROUND:

Angiotensin-converting-enzyme (ACE) inhibitors improve outcome of patients with chronic heart failure (CHF). A substantial proportion of patients, however, experience no benefit from ACE inhibitors because of previous intolerance. We aimed to find out whether candesartan, an angiotensin-receptor blocker, could improve outcome in such patients not taking an ACE inhibitor.

METHODS:

Between March, 1999, and March, 2001, we enrolled 2028 patients with symptomatic heart failure and left-ventricular ejection fraction 40% or less who were not receiving ACE inhibitors because of previous intolerance. Patients were randomly assigned candesartan (target dose 32 mg once daily) or matching placebo. The primary outcome of the study was the composite of cardiovascular death or hospital admission for CHF. Analysis was by intention to treat.

FINDINGS:

The most common manifestation of ACE-inhibitor intolerance was cough (72%), followed by symptomatic hypotension (13%) and renal dysfunction (12%). During a median follow-up of 33.7 months, 334 (33%) of 1013 patients in the candesartan group and 406 (40%) of 1015 in the placebo group had cardiovascular death or hospital admission for CHF (unadjusted hazard ratio 0.77 [95% CI 0.67-0.89], p=0.0004; covariate adjusted 0.70 [0.60-0.81], p<0.0001). Each component of the primary outcome was reduced, as was the total number of hospital admissions for CHF. Study-drug discontinuation rates were similar in the candesartan (30%) and placebo (29%) groups.

INTERPRETATION:

Candesartan was generally well tolerated and reduced cardiovascular mortality and morbidity in patients with symptomatic chronic heart failure and intolerance to ACE inhibitors.

RALES

THE EFFECT OF SPIRONOLACTONE ON MORBIDITY AND MORTALITY IN PATIENTS WITH SEVERE HEART FAILURE.
NEW ENGLAND JOURNAL OF MEDICINE (NEJM) 1999.

Rales was designed to investigate the effect of spironolactone on mortality in patients with severe symptomatic heart failure with reduced systolic function on optimal medical therapy. Patients were randomized to spironolactone or placebo. Treatment with spironolactone resulted in significant 30% lower all-cause mortality; it also lowered cardiac mortality from both progressive heart failure and sudden cardiac death.

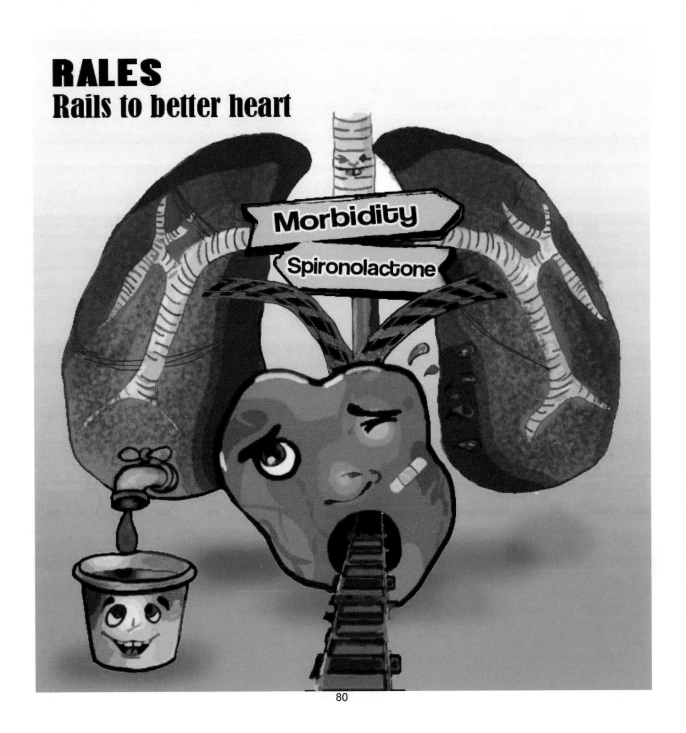

RALES

The effect of spironolactone on morbidity and mortality in patients with severe heart failure.

Pitt B, et al.

New England Journal of Medicine (NEJM) 1999; September 2;341(10):709-17

BACKGROUND AND METHODS:

Aldosterone is important in the pathophysiology of heart failure. In a double blind study, we enrolled 1663 patients who had severe heart failure and a left ventricular ejection fraction of no more than 35 percent and who were being treated with an angiotensin-converting-enzyme inhibitor, a loop diuretic, and in most cases digoxin. A total of 822 patients were randomly assigned to receive 25 mg of spironolactone daily, and 841 to receive placebo. The primary end point was death from all causes.

RESULTS:

The trial was discontinued early, after a mean follow-up period of 24 months, because an interim analysis determined that spironolactone was efficacious. There were 386 deaths in the placebo group (46 percent) and 284 in the spirono-lactone group (35 percent; relative risk of death, 0.70; 95 percent confidence interval, 0.60 to 0.82; $P<0.001$). This 30 percent reduction in the risk of death among patients in the spironolactone group was attributed to a lower risk of both death from progressive heart failure and sudden death from cardiac causes. The frequency of hospitalization for worsening heart failure was 35 percent lower in the spironolactone group than in the placebo group (relative risk of hospitalization, 0.65; 95 percent confidence interval, 0.54 to 0.77; $P<0.001$). In addition, patients who received spironolactone had a significant improvement in the symptoms of heart failure, as assessed on the basis of the New York Heart Association functional class ($P<0.001$). Gynecomastia or breast pain was reported in 10 percent of men who were treated with spironolactone, as compared with 1 percent of men in the placebo group ($P<0.001$). The incidence of serious hyperkalemia was minimal in both groups of patients.

CONCLUSIONS:

Blockade of aldosterone receptors by spironolactone, in addition to standard therapy, substantially reduces the risk of both morbidity and death among patients with severe heart failure.

EPHESUS

EPLERENONE, A SELECTIVE ALDOSTERONE BLOCKER, IN PATIENTS WITH LEFT VENTRICULAR DYSFUNCTION AFTER MYOCARDIAL INFARCTION.
NEW ENGLAND JOURNAL OF MEDICINE (NEJM) 2003.

EPHESUS trial was designed to evaluated eplerenone (a selective aldosterone blocker) effect on mortality and cardiovascular hospitalizations when added to optimal medical therapy in patients who suffered acute MI and resulted in cardiomyopathy, or history of diabetes if heart failure was not present. Patients treated with eplerenone had significant decrease in mortality. The mortality benefit was primarily driven by a reduction in sudden cardiac death.

Ephesus was an ancient Greek city, and later a major Roman city. It is Located in nowdays Turkey on the Mediterranean coast. Ephesus which was established as one of the most important ports, and commercial centers, was also an important center for early Christianity*.

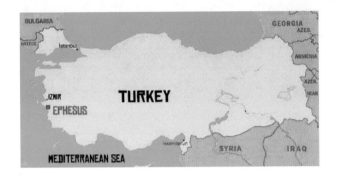

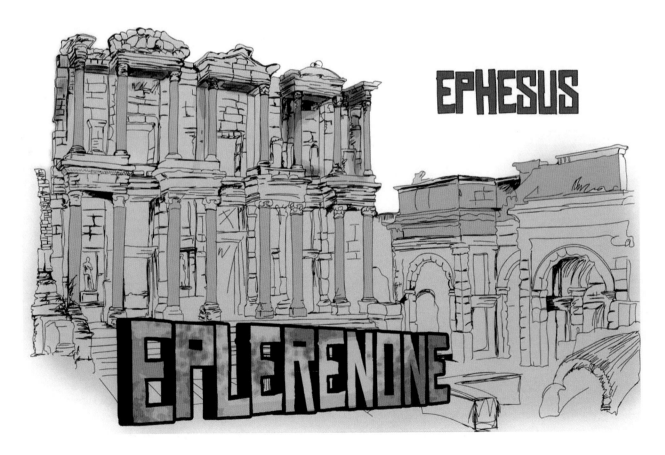

EPHESUS

Eplerenone, a selective aldosterone blocker, in patients with left ventricular dysfunction after myocardial infarction.

Pitt B, et al.

New England Journal of Medicine (NEJM) 2003; April 3; 348(14):1309-21.

BACKGROUND:

Aldosterone blockade reduces mortality and morbidity among patients with severe heart failure. We conducted a double-blind, placebo-controlled study evaluating the effect of eplerenone, a selective aldosterone blocker, on morbidity and mortality among patients with acute myocardial infarction complicated by left ventricular dysfunction and heart failure.

METHODS:

Patients were randomly assigned to eplerenone (25 mg per day initially, titrated to a maximum of 50 mg per day; 3319 patients) or placebo (3313 patients) in addition to optimal medical therapy. The study continued until 1012 deaths occurred. The primary end points were death from any cause and death from cardiovascular causes or hospitalization for heart failure, acute myocardial infarction, stroke, or ventricular arrhythmia.

RESULTS:

During a mean follow-up of 16 months, there were 478 deaths in the eplerenone group and 554 deaths in the placebo group (relative risk, 0.85; 95 percent confidence interval, 0.75 to 0.96; P=0.008). Of these deaths, 407 in the eplerenone group and 483 in the placebo group were attributed to cardiovascular causes (relative risk, 0.83; 95 percent confidence interval, 0.72 to 0.94; P=0.005). The rate of the other primary end point, death from cardiovascular causes or hospitalization for cardiovascular events, was reduced by eplerenone (relative risk, 0.87; 95 percent confidence interval, 0.79 to 0.95; P=0.002), as was the secondary end point of death from any cause or any hospitalization (relative risk, 0.92; 95 percent confidence interval, 0.86 to 0.98; P=0.02). There was also a reduction in the rate of sudden death from cardiac causes (relative risk, 0.79; 95 percent confidence interval, 0.64 to 0.97; P=0.03). The rate of serious hyperkalemia was 5.5 percent in the eplerenone group and 3.9 percent in the placebo group (P=0.002), whereas the rate of hypokalemia was 8.4 percent in the eplerenone group and 13.1 percent in the placebo group (P<0.001).

CONCLUSIONS:

The addition of eplerenone to optimal medical therapy reduces morbidity and mortality among patients with acute myocardial infarction complicated by left ventricular dysfunction and heart failure.

EMPHASIS-HF
Eplerenone in patients with systolic heart failure and mild symptoms.
Zannad F et al.
New England Journal of Medicine (NEJM) 2011; January 6; 364(1):11-21.

Emphasis-HF trial was designed to investigate the extension of use of aldosterone receptor antagonists in patients with mild heart failure symptoms and ejection fraction no more than 35%, patients were randomized to eplerenone or placebo in addition of optimal medical therapy. Patients treated with eplerenone had significant reduction in cardiovascular death and first heart failure hospitalization, the study was prematurely stopped due to the significantly higher events in the control group.

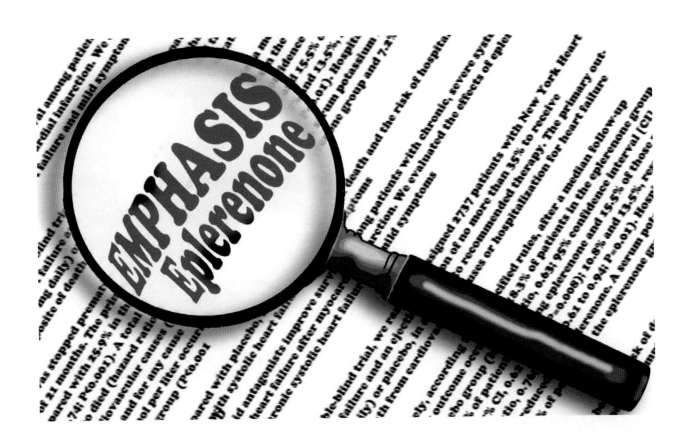

EMPHASIS-HF
Eplerenone in patients with systolic heart failure and mild symptoms.
Zannad F et al.
The New England Journal of Medicine (NEJM) 2011; January 6; 364(1):11-21.

BACKGROUND:

Mineralocorticoid antagonists improve survival among patients with chronic, severe systolic heart failure and heart failure after myocardial infarction. We evaluated the effects of eplerenone in patients with chronic systolic heart failure and mild symptoms.

METHODS:

In this randomized, double-blind trial, we randomly assigned 2737 patients with New York Heart Association class II heart failure and an ejection fraction of no more than 35% to receive eplerenone (up to 50 mg daily) or placebo, in addition to recommended therapy. The primary outcome was a composite of death from cardiovascular causes or hospitalization for heart failure.

RESULTS:

The trial was stopped prematurely, according to prespecified rules, after a median follow-up period of 21 months. The primary outcome occurred in 18.3% of patients in the eplerenone group as compared with 25.9% in the placebo group (hazard ratio, 0.63; 95% confidence interval [CI], 0.54 to 0.74; P<0.001). A total of 12.5% of patients receiving eplerenone and 15.5% of those receiving placebo died (hazard ratio, 0.76; 95% CI, 0.62 to 0.93; P=0.008); 10.8% and 13.5%, respectively, died of cardiovascular causes (hazard ratio, 0.76; 95% CI, 0.61 to 0.94; P=0.01). Hospitalizations for heart failure and for any cause were also reduced with eplerenone. A serum potassium level exceeding 5.5 mmol per liter occurred in 11.8% of patients in the eplerenone group and 7.2% of those in the placebo group (P<0.001).

CONCLUSIONS:

Eplerenone, as compared with placebo, reduced both the risk of death and the risk of hospitalization among patients with systolic heart failure and mild symptoms.

COPERNICUS
EFFECT OF CARVEDILOL ON SURVIVAL IN SEVERE CHRONIC HEART FAILURE
NEW ENGLAND JOURNAL OF MEDICINE (NEJM). 2001.

COPERNICUS trial aimed to evaluate effect of carvedilol on mortality in patients with severe heart failure and depressed LVEF. Patients randomized to carvedilol or placebo added to baseline medical therapy. After mean follow-up of about 10 months (study was terminated early), carvedilol significantly lowered mortality and hospitalization in all subgroups with fewer discontinuations in the carvedilol group. COPERNICUS extended the evidence that carvedilol lowers mortality even in patients with severe heart failure and recent decompensation.

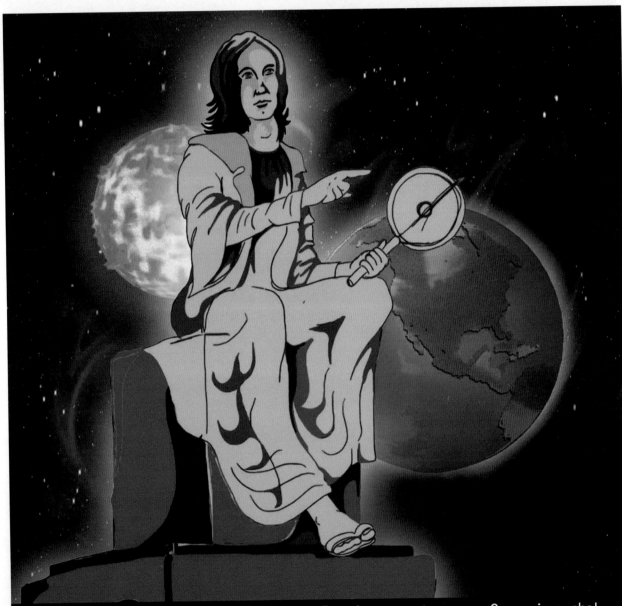

Nicolaus Copernicus (1473 – 1543) was a Renaissance astronomer, Copernicus challenged the traditional believes that the earth is the center of the universe, and proposed that the sun is the actual center of the universe. Whereas Copernicus trial challenged the notion that beta blocker with their negative inotropic effect suppose to be contraindicated in the decompnsated heart failure, and showed it is actually beneficial*.

*http://en.wikipedia.org

COPERNICUS

Effect of carvedilol on survival in severe chronic heart failure

Packer M, et al.

New England Journal of Medicine (NEJM). 2001; May 31; 344(22):1651-8.

BACKGROUND:

Beta-blocking agents reduce the risk of hospitalization and death in patients with mild-to-moderate heart failure, but little is known about their effects in severe heart failure.

METHODS:

We evaluated 2289 patients who had symptoms of heart failure at rest or on minimal exertion, who were clinically euvolemic, and who had an ejection fraction of less than 25 percent. In a double-blind fashion, we randomly assigned 1133 patients to placebo and 1156 patients to treatment with carvedilol for a mean period of 10.4 months, during which standard therapy for heart failure was continued. Patients who required intensive care, had marked fluid retention, or were receiving intravenous vasodilators or positive inotropic drugs were excluded.

RESULTS:

There were 190 deaths in the placebo group and 130 deaths in the carvedilol group. This difference reflected a 35 percent decrease in the risk of death with carvedilol (95 percent confidence interval, 19 to 48 percent; $P=0.00013$, unadjusted; $P=0.0014$, adjusted for interim analyses). A total of 507 patients died or were hospitalized in the placebo group, as compared with 425 in the carvedilol group. This difference reflected a 24 percent decrease in the combined risk of death or hospitalization with carvedilol (95 percent confidence interval, 13 to 33 percent; $P<0.001$). The favorable effects on both end points were seen consistently in all the subgroups we examined, including patients with a history of recent or recurrent cardiac decompensation. Fewer patients in the carvedilol group than in the placebo group withdrew because of adverse effects or for other reasons ($P=0.02$).

CONCLUSIONS:

The previously reported benefits of carvedilol with regard to morbidity and mortality in patients with mild-to-moderate heart failure were also apparent in the patients with severe heart failure who were evaluated in this trial.

CAPRICORN was one of the early trials to evaluate the benefit of Carvedilol in patients with systolic dysfunction after myocardial infarction. Although the study was statistically negative (p=0.031 >0.005), patients who were randomized to carvedilol showed 23% reduction in all cause mortality, and less recurrent non-fatal myocardial infarctions. While the US Carvedilol study, which included patients with CHF and decreased LVEF, was terminated early after the result showing that there was significant reduction in mortality and morbidity in patients receiving carvedilol versus placebo.

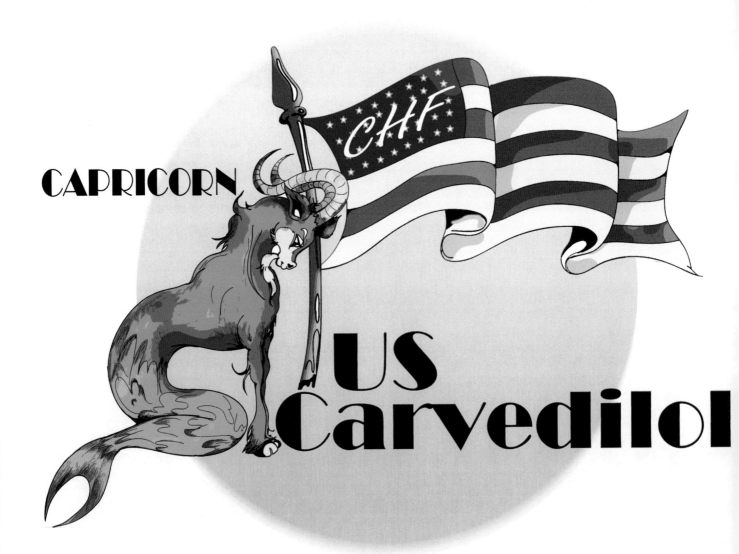

CAPRICORN

US Carvedilol

US CARVIDOLOL TRIAL

The effect of carvedilol on morbidity and mortality in patients with chronic heart failure. Packer M, et al.

New England Journal of Medicine (NEJM). 1996 May 23;334(21):1349-55.

BACKGROUND:

Controlled clinical trials have shown that beta-blockers can produce hemodynamic and symptomatic improvement in chronic heart failure, but the effect of these drugs on survival has not been determined.

METHODS:

We enrolled 1094 patients with chronic heart failure in a double-blind, placebo-controlled, stratified program, in which patients were assigned to one of the four treatment protocols on the basis of their exercise capacity. Within each of the four protocols patients with mild, moderate, or severe heart failure with left ventricular ejection fractions < or = 0.35 were randomly assigned to receive either placebo (n = 398) or the beta-blockercarvedilol (n = 696); background therapy with digoxin, diuretics, and an angiotensin-converting-enzyme inhibitor remained constant. Patient were observed for the occurrence death or hospitalization for cardiovascular reasons during the following 6 months, after the beginning (12 months for the group with mild heart failure).

RESULTS:

The overall mortality rate was 7.8 percent in the placebo group and 3.2 percent in the carvedilol group; the reduction in risk attributable tocarvedilol was 65 percent (95 percent confidence interval, 39 to 80 percent; P < 0.001). This finding led the Data and Safety Monitoring Board to recommend termination of the study before its scheduled completion. In addition, as compared with placebo, carvedilol therapy was accompanied by a 27 percent reduction in the risk of hospitalization for cardiovascular causes (19.6 percent vs. 14.1 percent, P = 0.036), as well as a 38 percent reduction in the combined risk of hospitalization or death (24.6 percent vs, 15.8 percent, P < 0.001). Worsening heart failure as an adverse reaction during treatment was less frequent in the carvedilol than in the placebo group.

CONCLUSIONS:

Carvedilol reduces the risk or death as well as the risk of hospitalization for cardiovascular causes in patients with heart failure who are receiving treatment with digoxin, diuretics, and an angiotensin-converting-enzyme inhibitor.

CAPRICORN TRIAL

Effect of carvedilol on outcome after myocardial infarction in patients with left-ventricular dysfunction Dargie HJ. et al.

Lancet. 2001 May 5;357(9266):1385-90

BACKGROUND:

The beneficial effects of beta-blockers on long-term outcome after acute myocardial infarction were shown before the introduction of thrombolysis and angiotensin-converting-enzyme (ACE) inhibitors. Generally, the patients recruited to these trials were at low risk: few had heart failure, and none had measurements of left-ventricular function taken. We investigated the long-term efficacy of carvedilol on morbidity and mortality in patients with left-ventricular dysfunction after acute myocardial infarction treated according to current evidence-based practice.

METHODS:

In a multicentre, randomised, placebo-controlled trial, 1959 patients with a proven acute myocardial infarction and a left-ventricular ejection fraction of </=40% were randomly assigned 6.25 mg carvedilol (n=975) or placebo (n=984). Study medication was progressively increased to a maximum of 25 mg twice daily during the next 4-6 weeks, and patients were followed up until the requisite number of primary endpoints had occurred. The primary endpoint was all-cause mortality or hospital admission for cardiovascular problems. Analysis was by intention to treat.

FINDINGS:

Although there was no difference between the carvedilol and placebo groups in the number of patients with the primary endpoint (340 [35%] vs 367 [37%], hazard ratio 0.92 [95% CI 0.80-1.07]), all-cause mortality alone was lower in the carvedilol group than in the placebo group (116 [12%] vs. 151 [15%], 0.77 [0.60-0.98], p=0.03). Cardiovascular mortality, non-fatal myocardial infarctions, and all-cause mortality or non-fatal myocardial infarction were also lower on carvedilol than on placebo.

INTERPRETATION:

In patients treated long-term after an acute myocardial infarction complicated by left ventricular systolic dysfunction, carvedilol reduced the frequency of all-cause and cardiovascular mortality, and recurrent, non-fatal myocardial infarctions. These beneficial effects are additional to those of evidence-based treatments for acute myocardial infarction including ACE inhibitors

COMET TRIAL

COMPARISON OF CARVEDILOL AND METOPROLOL ON CLINICAL OUTCOMES IN PATIENTS WITH CHRONIC HEART FAILURE IN THE CARVEDILOL OR METOPROLOL EUROPEAN TRIAL
POOLE-WILSON PA ET AL. CARVEDILOL OR METOPROLOL EUROPEAN TRIAL INVESTIGATORS.
LANCET. 2003; JULY 5; 362(9377):7-13

COMET was designed to directly compare two beta blockers in the treatment of symptomatic chronic heart failure and reduced systolic function. Patients in COMET were randomized to either carvedilol or metoprolol tartrate. It showed significant 17% reduction in the relative risk of all-cause death in group treated with carvedilol compared to metoprolol tartrate.

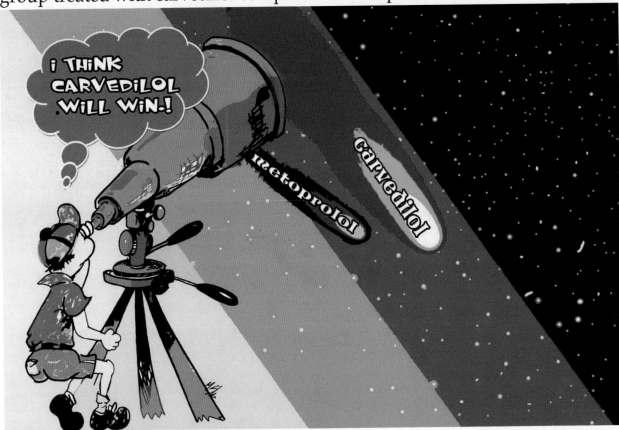

BACKGROUND: Beta blockers reduce mortality in patients who have chronic heart failure, systolic dysfunction, and are on background treatment with diuretics and angiotensin-converting enzyme inhibitors. We aimed to compare the effects of carvedilol and metoprolol on clinical outcome.

METHODS: In a multicentre, double-blind, and randomised parallel group trial, we assigned 1511 patients with chronic heart failure to treatment with carvedilol (target dose 25 mg twice daily) and 1518 to metoprolol (metoprolol tartrate, target dose 50 mg twice daily). Patients were required to have chronic heart failure (NYHA II-IV), previous admission for a cardiovascular reason, an ejection fraction of less than 0.35, and to have been treated optimally with diuretics and angiotensin-converting enzyme inhibitors unless not tolerated. The primary endpoints were all-cause mortality and the composite endpoint of all-cause mortality or all-cause admission. Analysis was done by intention to treat.

FINDINGS: The mean study duration was 58 months (SD 6). The mean ejection fraction was 0.26 (0.07) and the mean age 62 years (11). The all-cause mortality was 34% (512 of 1511) for carvedilol and 40% (600 of 1518) for metoprolol (hazard ratio 0.83 [95% CI 0.74-0.93], p=0.0017). The reduction of all-cause mortality was consistent across predefined subgroups. The composite endpoint of mortality or all-cause admission occurred in 1116 (74%) of 1511 on carvedilol and in 1160 (76%) of 1518 on metoprolol (0.94 [0.86-1.02], p=0.122). Incidence of side-effects and drug withdrawals did not differ by much between the two study groups.

INTERPRETATION: Our results suggest that carvedilol extends survival compared with metoprolol.

V-HEFT AND A-HEFT TRAILS

V-HEFT was the first trial to show the benefit of the combination of Hydralazine and Nitrate in Heart Failure. Actually V-HEFT was the first heart failure trial to be powered to show a mortality benefit, and a subgroup analysis of V-HeFT suggested that African American patients may have more benefit from this combination, so the A-HEFT trial was conducted and showed the benefit of a fixed dose of Hydralazine and Nitrate in African American patients. A-HeFT led to the first racially indicated FDA approval of a drug!\

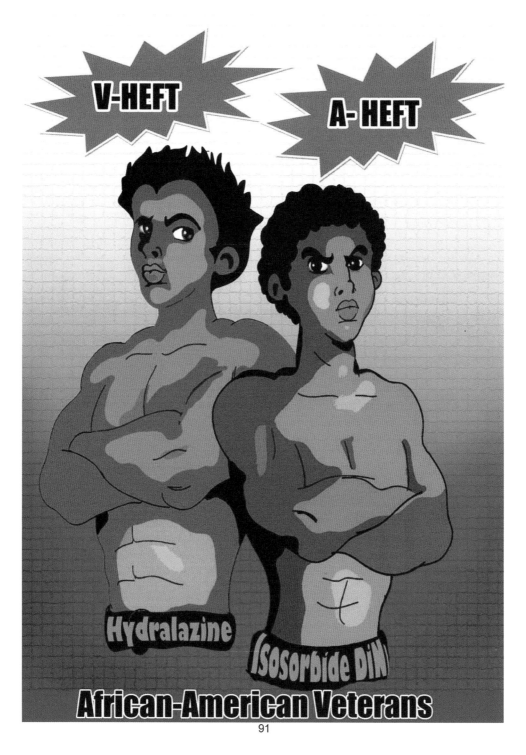

V-Heft TRAIL

Effect of vasodilator therapy on mortality in chronic congestive heart failure.
Results of a Veterans Administration Cooperative Study. Cohn JN, et al.

New England Journal of Medicine (NEJM). 1986 June 12;314(24):1547-52.

To evaluate the effects of vasodilator therapy on mortality among patients with chronic congestive heart failure, we randomly assigned 642 men with impaired cardiac function and reduced exercise tolerance who were taking digoxin and a diuretic to receive additional double-blind treatment with placebo, prazosin (20 mg per day), or the combination of hydralazine (300 mg per day) and isosorbide dinitrate (160 mg per day). Follow-up averaged 2.3 years (range, 6 months to 5.7 years). Mortality over the entire follow-up period was lower in the group that received hydralazine and isosorbide dinitrate than in the placebo group. This difference was of borderline statistical significance. For mortality by two years, a major end point specified in the protocol, the risk reduction among patients treated with both hydralazine and isosorbide dinitrate was 34 percent (P less than 0.028). The cumulative mortality rates at two years were 25.6 percent in the hydralazine--isosorbide dinitrate group and 34.3 percent in the placebo group; at three years, the mortality rate was 36.2 percent versus 46.9 percent. The mortality-risk reduction in the group treated with hydralazine and isosorbide dinitrate was 36 percent by three years. The mortality in the prazosin group was similar to that in the placebo group. Left ventricular ejection fraction (measured sequentially) rose significantly at eight weeks and at one year in the group treated with hydralazine and isosorbide dinitrate but not in the placebo or prazosin groups. Our data suggest that the addition of hydralazine and isosorbide dinitrate to the therapeutic regimen of digoxin and diuretics in patients with chronic congestive heart failure can have a favorable effect on left ventricular function and mortality.

A- HEFT TRIAL

Combination of isosorbide dinitrate and hydralazine in blacks with heart failure.
Taylor AL, et al. African-American Heart Failure Trial Investigators

New England Journal of Medicine (NEJM) . 2004; November 11; 351(20):2049-57.

BACKGROUND:
We examined whether a fixed dose of both isosorbide dinitrate and hydralazine provides additional benefit in blacks with advanced heart failure, a subgroup previously noted to have a favorable response to this therapy.

METHODS:
A total of 1050 black patients who had New York Heart Association class III or IV heart failure with dilated ventricles were randomly assigned to receive a fixed dose of isosorbide dinitrate plus hydralazine or placebo in addition to standard therapy for heart failure. The primary end point was a composite score made up of weighted values for death from any cause, a first hospitalization for heart failure, and change in the quality of life.

RESULTS:
The study was terminated early owing to a significantly higher mortality rate in the placebo group than in the group given isosorbide dinitrate plus hydralazine (10.2 percent vs. 6.2 percent, P=0.02). The mean primary composite score was significantly better in the group given isosorbide dinitrate plus hydralazine than in the placebo group (-0.1+/-1.9 vs. -0.5+/-2.0, P=0.01; range of possible values, -6 to +2), as were its individual components (43 percent reduction in the rate of death from any cause [hazard ratio, 0.57; P=0.01] 33 percent relative reduction in the rate of first hospitalization for heart failure [16.4 percent vs. 22.4 percent, P=0.001], and an improvement in the quality of life [change in score, -5.6+/-20.6 vs. -2.7+/-21.2, with lower scores indicating better quality of life; P=0.02; range of possible values, 0 to 105]).

CONCLUSIONS:
The addition of a fixed dose of isosorbide dinitrate plus hydralazine to standard therapy for heart failure including neurohormonal blockers is efficacious and increases survival among black patients with advanced heart failure.

VMAC TRIAL
INTRAVENOUS NESIRITIDE VS NITROGLYCERIN FOR TREATMENT OF DECOMPENSATED CONGESTIVE HEART FAILURE: A RANDOMIZED CONTROLLED TRIAL.
JOURNAL OF THE AMERICAN MEDICAL ASSOCIATION (JAMA). 2002 MARCH 27;287(12):1531-40.

VMAC established the rule that IV vasodilators may play in the acute management of heart Failure. While IV nitroglycerin, which is widely used, showed only a trend to improvement in PWCP with no symptomatic improvement (on small doses). On the other hand nesiritide showed a better PWCP reduction and mild symptomatic improvement over placebo and nitroglycerin.

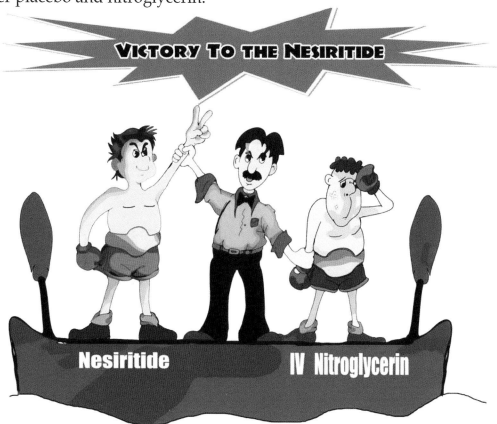

CONTEXT: Decompensated congestive heart failure (CHF) is the leading hospital discharge diagnosis in patients older than 65 years.

OBJECTIVE: To compare the efficacy and safety of intravenous nesiritide, intravenous nitroglycerin, and placebo.

DESIGN, SETTING, AND PATIENTS: Randomized, double-blind trial of 489 inpatients with dyspnea at rest from decompensated CHF, including 246 who received pulmonary artery catheterization, that was conducted at 55 community and academic hospitals between October 1999 and July 2000.

INTERVENTIONS: Intravenous nesiritide (n = 204), intravenous nitroglycerin (n = 143), or placebo (n = 142) added to standard medications for 3 hours, followed by nesiritide (n = 278) or nitroglycerin (n = 216) added to standard medication for 24 hours.

MAIN OUTCOME MEASURES: Change in pulmonary capillary wedge pressure (PCWP) among catheterized patients and patient self-evaluation of dyspnea at 3 hours after initiation of study drug among all patients. Secondary outcomes included comparisons of hemodynamic and clinical effects between nesiritide and nitroglycerin at 24 hours.

RESULTS: At 3 hours, the mean (SD) decrease in PCWP from baseline was -5.8 (6.5) mm Hg for nesiritide (vs placebo, P<.001; vs nitroglycerin, P =.03), -3.8 (5.3) mm Hg for nitroglycerin (vs placebo, P =.09), and -2 (4.2) mm Hg for placebo. At 3 hours, nesiritide resulted in improvement in dyspnea compared with placebo (P =.03), but there was no significant difference in dyspnea or global clinical status with nesiritide compared with nitroglycerin. At 24 hours, the reduction in PCWP was greater in the nesiritide group (-8.2 mm Hg) than the nitroglycerin group (-6.3 mm Hg), but patients reported no significant differences in dyspnea and only modest improvement in global clinical status.

CONCLUSION: When added to standard care in patients hospitalized with acutely decompensated CHF, nesiritide improves hemodynamic function and some self-reported symptoms more effectively than intravenous nitroglycerin or placebo.

FUSION II TRIAL
SAFETY AND EFFICACY OF OUTPATIENT NESIRITIDE IN PATIENTS WITH ADVANCED HEART FAILURE
CIRCULATION HEART FAILURE . 2008.

As VAMC showed potential benefit of nesiritide in the setting of acute heart failure; FUSION-II tried to see whether using nesiritide as outpatient infusion will offer benefit in patients with advanced heart failure. However nesiritide failed to show any reduction in either the rates of death or hospitalization.

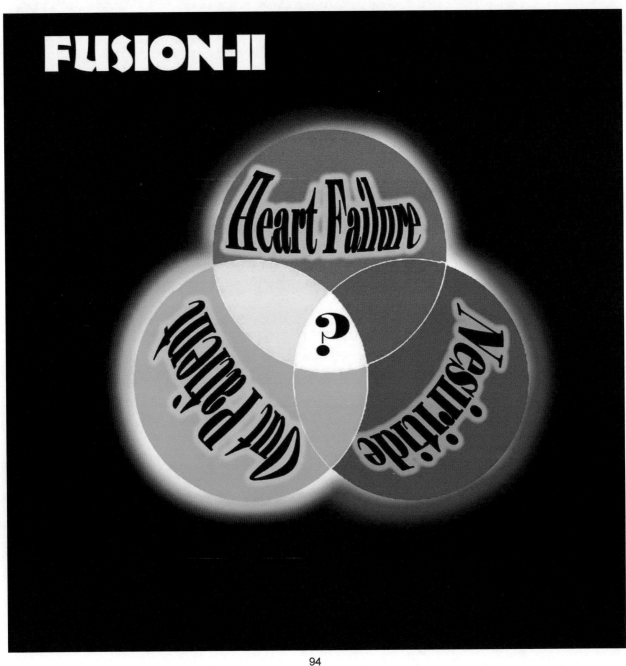

FUSION II TRIAL

Safety and efficacy of outpatient nesiritide in patients with advanced heart failure: results of the Second Follow-Up Serial Infusions of Nesiritide (FUSION II) trial.

Yancy CW, et al.

Circulation Heart failure. 2008; May; 1(1):9-16.

BACKGROUND:

Patients with American College of Cardiology/American Heart Association stage C/D heart failure experience substantial morbidity and mortality, but available interventions beyond standard medical and device therapies are limited. Nesiritide relieves dyspnea and reduces pulmonary congestion, but its risk profile is uncertain. Pilot data suggested a potential benefit of nesiritide given as serial outpatient infusions.

METHODS AND RESULTS:

The Second Follow-Up Serial Infusions of Nesiritide (FUSION II) trial was a randomized, double-blind, placebo-controlled trial of outpatient serial nesiritide infusions for patients with American College of Cardiology/American Heart Association stage C/D heart failure. Patients with 2 recent heart failure hospitalizations, ejection fraction <40%, and New York Heart Association class IV symptoms, or New York Heart Association class III symptoms with creatinine clearance <60 mL/min, were randomized to nesiritide (2-microg/kg bolus plus 0.01-microg/kg-per-minute infusion for 4 to 6 hours) or matching placebo, once or twice weekly for 12 weeks. All patients were treated to optimal goals with evidence-based medical/device therapy facilitated by careful disease management during the study. The primary end point was time to all-cause death or cardiovascular or renal hospitalization at 12 weeks. A total of 911 patients were randomized and treated. The primary end point occurred in 36.8% and 36.7% of the placebo and nesiritide groups, respectively (hazard ratio, 1.03; 95% confidence interval, 0.82 to 1.3; log-rank test P=0.79). There were no statistically significant differences between groups in any of the secondary end points, including the number of cardiovascular or renal hospitalizations, the number of days alive and out of the hospital, change in Kansas City Cardiomyopathy Questionnaire score, or cardiovascular death. Adverse events were similar between groups; nesiritide was associated with more hypotension but less predefined worsening renal function.

CONCLUSIONS:

Serial outpatient nesiritide infusions do not provide a demonstrable clinical benefit over intensive outpatient management of patients with advanced American College of Cardiology/American Heart Association stage C/D heart failure.

OPTIME-CHF TRIAL

SHORT-TERM INTRAVENOUS MILRINONE FOR ACUTE EXACERBATION OF CHRONIC HEART FAILURE: A RANDOMIZED CONTROLLED TRIAL.
JOURNAL OF THE AMERICAN MEDICAL ASSOCIATION (JAMA). 2002.

OPTIME- CHF trial looked at the potential benefit of using intravenous inotropic therapy (milrinone) in patients hospitalized with heart failure symptoms. However, patients who were treated with milrinone showed increased atrial arrhythmias and sustained hypotension with no significant difference of the hospitalization rate between the two groups. The results were not in favor of using milrinone routinely in this patients population.

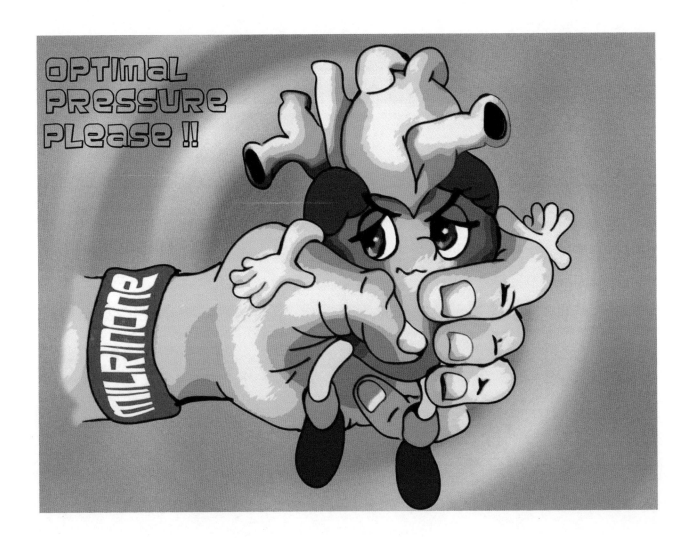

OPTIME-CHF TRIAL

Short-term intravenous milrinone for acute exacerbation of chronic heart failure: a randomized controlled trial.

Cuffe MS, et al. Outcomes of a Prospective Trial of Intravenous Milrinone for Exacerbations of Chronic Heart Failure (OPTIME-CHF) Investigators.

Journal of the American Medical Association. 2002; March 27; 287(12):1541-7.

CONTEXT:

Little randomized evidence is available to guide the in-hospital management of patients with an acute exacerbation of chronic heart failure. Although intravenous inotropic therapy usually produces beneficial hemodynamic effects and is labeled for use in the care of such patients, the effect of such therapy on intermediate-term clinical outcomes is uncertain.

OBJECTIVE:

To prospectively test whether a strategy that includes short-term use of milrinone in addition to standard therapy can improve clinical outcomes of patients hospitalized with an exacerbation of chronic heart failure.

DESIGN:

Prospective, randomized, double-blind, placebo-controlled trial conducted from July 1997 through November 1999.

SETTING:

Seventy-eight community and tertiary care hospitals in the United States.

PARTICIPANTS:

A total of 951 patients admitted with an exacerbation of systolic heart failure not requiring intravenous inotropic support (mean age, 65 years; 92% with baseline New York Heart Association class III or IV; mean left ventricular ejection fraction, 23%).

INTERVENTION:

Patients were randomly assigned to receive a 48-hour infusion of either milrinone, 0.5 microg/kg per minute initially (n = 477), or saline placebo (n = 472).

MAIN OUTCOME MEASURE:

Cumulative days of hospitalization for cardiovascular cause within 60 days following randomization.

RESULTS:

The median number of days hospitalized for cardiovascular causes within 60 days after randomization did not differ significantly between patients given milrinone (6 days) compared with placebo (7 days; P =.71). Sustained hypotension requiring intervention (10.7% vs 3.2%; P<.001) and new atrial arrhythmias (4.6% vs 1.5%; P =.004) occurred more frequently in patients who received milrinone. The milrinone and placebo groups did not differ significantly in in-hospital mortality (3.8% vs 2.3%; P =.19), 60-day mortality (10.3% vs 8.9%; P =.41), or the composite incidence of death or readmission (35.0% vs 35.3%; P =.92)

CONCLUSION:

These results do not support the routine use of intravenous milrinone as an adjunct to standard therapy in the treatment of patients hospitalized for an exacerbation of chronic heart failure.

BNP AND TIME- CHF TRIALS

The utility of the B-type-natriuretic peptide (BNP) in the diagnosis and management of patients with CHF was tested in a number of clinical trials.BNP Trial established the benefit of using rapid BNP testing in the emergency department to help differentiate cardiac from pulmonary etiologies of dyspnea; a widely utilized practice nowadays. Off note, patients with Cor Pulmonale had also high level of BNP compared to other patients with pulmonary causes of dyspnea. The TIME-CHF trail tried to see whether a BNP-Guided therapy would be of more benefit than symptoms-guided therapy in the management of patients with CHF. TIME-CHF failed to show any clinical or quality of life benefits when using BNP levels as a marker for therapy over symptom-guided treatment.

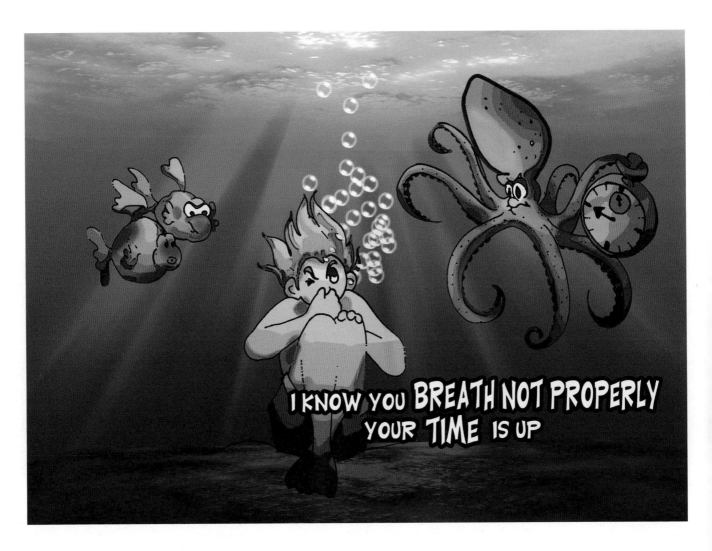

Breath Not Properly (BNP) TRIAL

Utility of a rapid B-natriuretic peptide assay in differentiating congestive heart failure from lung disease in patients presenting with dyspnea.
Morrison LK, et al.

The American College of Cardiology. 2002; January 16; 39(2):202-9.

OBJECTIVES:
Since B-type natriuretic peptide (BNP) is secreted by the left ventricle (LV) in response to volume elevated LV pressure, we sought to assess whether a rapid assay for BNP levels could differentiate cardiac from pulmonary causes of dyspnea.

BACKGROUND:
Differentiating congestive heart failure (CHF) from pulmonary causes of dyspnea is very important for patients presenting to the emergency department (ED) with acute dyspnea.

METHODS: B-natriuretic peptide levels were obtained in 321 patients presenting to the ED with acute dyspnea. Physicians were blinded to BNP levels and asked to give their probability of the patient having CHF and their final diagnosis. Two independent cardiologists were blinded to BNP levels and asked to review the data and evaluate which patients presented with heart failure. Patients with right heart failure from cor pulmonale were classified as having CHF.

RESULTS: Patients with CHF (n = 134) had BNP levels of 758.5 +/- 798 pg/ml, significantly higher than the group of patients with a final diagnosis of pulmonary disease (n = 85) whose BNP was 61 +/- 10 pg/ml. The area under the receiver operating curve, which plots sensitivity versus specificity for BNP levels in separating cardiac from pulmonary disease, was 0.96 (p < 0.001). A breakdown of patients with pulmonary disease revealed: chronic obstructive pulmonary disease (COPD): 54 +/- 71 pg/ml (n = 42); asthma: 27 +/- 40 pg/ml (n = 11); acute bronchitis: 44 +/- 112 pg/ml (n = 14); pneumonia: 55 +/- 76 pg/ml (n = 8); tuberculosis: 93 +/- 54 pg/ml (n = 2); lung cancer: 120 +/- 120 pg/ml (n = 4); and acute pulmonary embolism: 207 +/- 272 pg/ml (n = 3). In patients with a history of lung disease but whose current complaint of dyspnea was seen as due to CHF, BNP levels were 731 +/- 764 pg/ml (n = 54). The group with a history of CHF but with a current COPD diagnosis had a BNP of 47 +/- 23 pg/ml (n = 11).

CONCLUSIONS: Rapid testing of BNP in the ED should help differentiate pulmonary from cardiac etiologies of dyspnea.

TIME- CHF TRIAL

BNP-guided vs symptom-guided heart failure therapy: the Trial of Intensified vs Standard Medical Therapy in Elderly Patients With Congestive Heart Failure (TIME-CHF) randomized trial. Pfisterer M, et al.

Journal of the American Medical Association (JAMA). 2009; January 28; 301(4):383-92.

CONTEXT: It is uncertain whether intensified heart failure therapy guided by N-terminal brain natriuretic peptide (BNP) is superior to symptom-guided therapy.

OBJECTIVE: To compare 18-month outcomes of N-terminal BNP-guided vs symptom-guided heart failure therapy.

DESIGN, SETTING, AND PATIENTS:
Randomized controlled multicenter Trial of Intensified vs Standard Medical Therapy in Elderly Patients With Congestive Heart Failure (TIME-CHF) of 499 patients aged 60 years or older with systolic heart failure (ejection fraction < or = 45%), New York Heart Association (NYHA) class of II or greater, prior hospitalization for heart failure within 1 year, and N-terminal BNP level of 2 or more times the upper limit of normal. The study had an 18-month follow-up and it was conducted at 15 outpatient centers in Switzerland and Germany between January 2003 and June 2008.

INTERVENTION: Uptitration of guideline-based treatments to reduce symptoms to NYHA class of II or less (symptom-guided therapy) and BNP level of 2 times or less the upper limit of normal and symptoms to NYHA class of II or less (BNP-guided therapy).

MAIN OUTCOME MEASURES:
Primary outcomes were 18-month survival free of all-cause hospitalizations and quality of life as assessed by structured validated questionnaires.

RESULTS: Heart failure therapy guided by N-terminal BNP and symptom-guided therapy resulted in similar rates of survival free of all-cause hospitalizations (41% vs 40%, respectively; hazard ratio [HR], 0.91 [95% CI, 0.72-1.14]; P = .39). Patients' quality-of-life metrics improved over 18 months of follow-up but these improvements were similar in both the N-terminal BNP-guided and symptom-guided strategies. Compared with the symptom-guided group, survival free of hospitalization for heart failure, a secondary end point, was higher among those in the N-terminal BNP-guided group (72% vs 62%, respectively; HR, 0.68 [95% CI, 0.50-0.92]; P = .01). Heart failure therapy guided by N-terminal BNP improved outcomes in patients aged 60 to 75 years but not in those aged 75 years or older (P < .02 for interaction)

CONCLUSION: Heart failure therapy guided by N-terminal BNP did not improve overall clinical outcomes or quality of life compared with symptom-guided treatment.

IMPROVE-CHF

N-TERMINAL PRO-B-TYPE NATRIURETIC PEPTIDE TESTING IMPROVES THE MANAGEMENT OF PATIENTS WITH SUSPECTED ACUTE HEART FAILURE: PRIMARY RESULTS OF THE CANADIAN PROSPECTIVE RANDOMIZED MULTICENTER IMPROVE-CHF STUDY.
MOE GW, ET AL.
CANADIAN MULTICENTER IMPROVED MANAGEMENT OF PATIENTS WITH CONGESTIVE HEART FAILURE (IMPROVE-CHF) STUDY INVESTIGATORS.
CIRCULATION. 2007; JUNE 19; 115(24):3103-10.

While BNP trial established the utility of using BNP in ER in diagnosing cardiac causes of CHF. IMPROVE-CHF established the benefit of comparing subsequent BNP in ER presentation not only improving diagnostic capabilities, but also in improving patients' outcomes, reducing the duration of ED visit, and cutting healthcare cost.

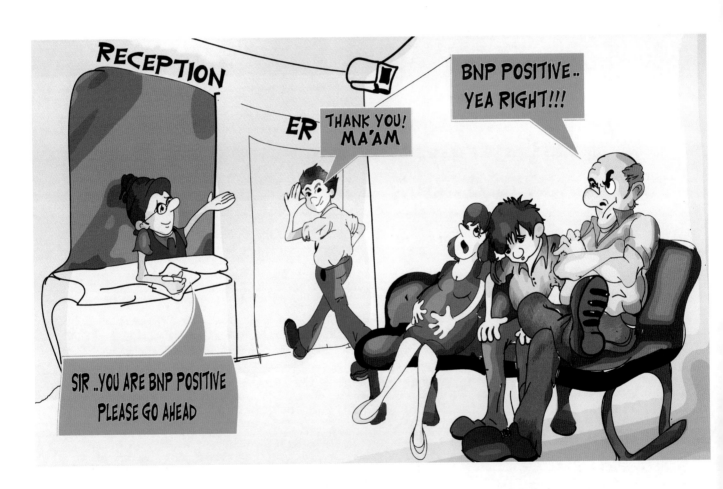

IMPROVE-CHF

N-terminal pro-B-type natriuretic peptide testing improves the management of patients with suspected acute heart failure: primary results of the Canadian prospective randomized multicenter IMPROVE-CHF study.

Moe GW, et al.

Canadian Multicenter Improved Management of Patients With Congestive Heart Failure (IMPROVE-CHF) Study Investigators.

Circulation. 2007; June 19; 115(24):3103-10.

BACKGROUND:

The diagnostic utility of N-terminal pro-B-type natriuretic peptide (NT-proBNP) in heart failure has been documented. However, most of the data were derived from countries with high healthcare resource use, and randomized evidence for utility of NT-proBNP was lacking.

METHODS AND RESULTS:

We tested the hypothesis that NT-proBNP testing improves the management of patients presenting with dyspnea to emergency departments in Canada by prospectively comparing the clinical and economic impact of a randomized management strategy either guided by NT-proBNP results or without knowledge of NT-proBNP concentrations. Five hundred patients presenting with dyspnea to 7 emergency departments were studied. The median NT-proBNP level among the 230 subjects with a final diagnosis of heart failure was 3697 compared with 212 pg/mL in those without heart failure ($P<0.00001$). Knowledge of NT-proBNP results reduced the duration of ED visit by 21% (6.3 to 5.6 hours; $P=0.031$), the number of patients rehospitalized over 60 days by 35% (51 to 33; $P=0.046$), and direct medical costs of all ED visits, hospitalizations, and subsequent outpatient services (US $6129 to US $5180 per patient; $P=0.023$) over 60 days from enrollment. Adding NT-proBNP to clinical judgment enhanced the accuracy of a diagnosis; the area under the receiver-operating characteristic curve increased from 0.83 to 0.90 ($P<0.00001$).

CONCLUSIONS:

In a universal health coverage system mandating judicious use of healthcare resources, inclusion of NT-proBNP testing improves the management of patients presenting to emergency departments with dyspnea through improved diagnosis, cost savings, and improvement in selected outcomes.

UNLOAD TRAIL

ULTRAFILTRATION VERSUS INTRAVENOUS DIURETICS FOR PATIENTS HOSPITALIZED FOR ACUTE DE-COMPENSATED HEART FAILURE.

JOURNAL OF THE AMERICAN COLLEGE OF CARDIOLOGY (JACC) 2007.

UNLOAD trial was the first trial to establish the potential benefit of ultrafiltration (UF) in the management of CHF. UNLOAD showed that UF was associated with significant weight and fluid loss when compared to standard diuretics therapy. Also UF was associated with decrease in both hospitalization rates and length of stay. However there was no significant difference in either symptoms relief or renal function in this trial.

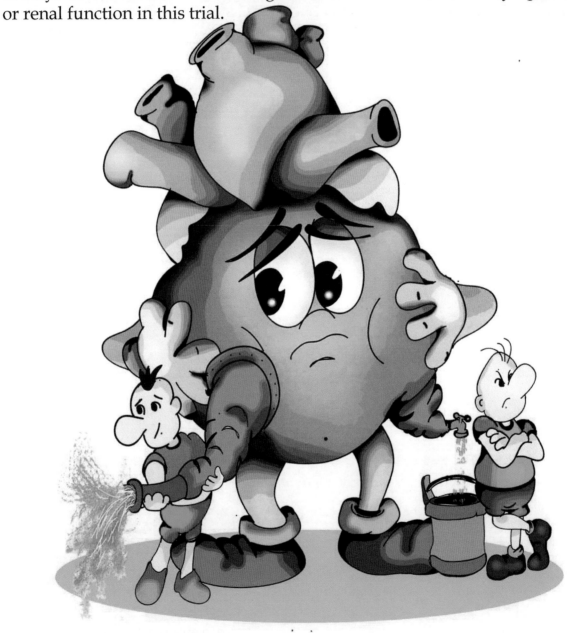

Ultrafiltration Versus Intravenous Diuretics

UNLOAD TRAIL

Ultrafiltration versus intravenous diuretics for patients hospitalized for acute decompensated heart failure.

Costanzo MR, et al. UNLOAD Trial Investigators.

Journal of the American College of Cardiology (JACC) 2007; February 13; 49(6):675-83.

OBJECTIVES:

This study was designed to compare the safety and efficacy of veno-venous ultrafiltration and standard intravenous diuretic therapy for hypervolemic heart failure (HF) patients.

BACKGROUND:

Early ultrafiltration may be an alternative to intravenous diuretics in patients with decompensated HF and volume overload.

METHODS:

Patients hospitalized for HF with > or =2 signs of hypervolemia were randomized to ultrafiltration or intravenous diuretics. Primary end points were weight loss and dyspnea assessment at 48 h after randomization. Secondary end points included net fluid loss at 48 h, functional capacity, HF rehospitalizations, and unscheduled visits in 90 days. Safety end points included changes in renal function, electrolytes, and blood pressure.

RESULTS:

Two hundred patients (63 +/- 15 years, 69% men, 71% ejection fraction < or =40%) were randomized to ultrafiltration or intravenous diuretics. At 48 h, weight (5.0 +/- 3.1 kg vs. 3.1 +/- 3.5 kg; p = 0.001) and net fluid loss (4.6 vs. 3.3 l; p = 0.001) were greater in the ultrafiltration group. Dyspnea scores were similar. At 90 days, the ultrafiltration group had fewer patients rehospitalized for HF (16 of 89 [18%] vs. 28 of 87 [32%]; p = 0.037), HF rehospitalizations (0.22 +/- 0.54 vs. 0.46 +/- 0.76; p = 0.022), rehospitalization days (1.4 +/- 4.2 vs. 3.8 +/- 8.5; p = 0.022) per patient, and unscheduled visits (14 of 65 [21%] vs. 29 of 66 [44%]; p = 0.009). No serum creatinine differences occurred between groups. Nine deaths occurred in the ultrafiltration group and 11 in the diuretics group.

CONCLUSIONS:

In decompensated HF, ultrafiltration safely produces greater weight and fluid loss than intravenous diuretics, reduces 90-day resource utilization for HF, and is an effective alternative therapy.

ESCAPE TRIAL

EVALUATION STUDY OF CONGESTIVE HEART FAILURE AND PULMONARY ARTERY CATHETERIZATION EFFECTIVENESS: THE ESCAPE TRIAL.
JOURNAL OF THE AMERICAN MEDICAL ASSOCIATION (JAMA). 2005.

ESCAPE Trial was done to see the possible benefit in utilization of the pulmonary artery catheter (PAC) (the Swan-Ganz catheter)in guiding management of patients hospitalized with CHF. However, the Swan Ganz-catheter-guided therapy failed to show any benefit over management guided by clinical assessment, and was associated with more adverse events..

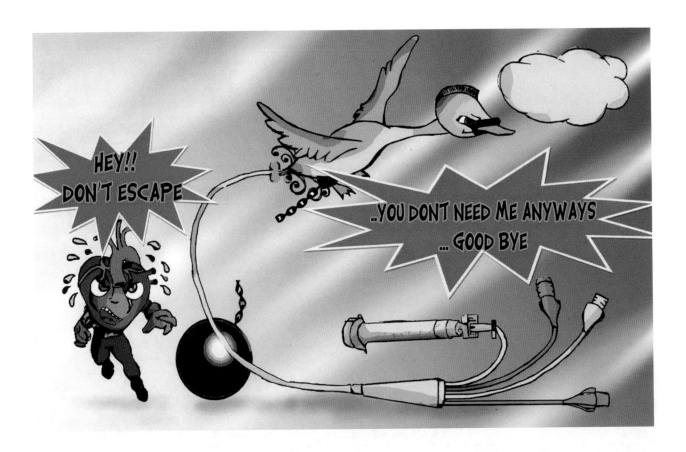

ESCAPE TRIAL

Evaluation study of congestive heart failure and pulmonary artery catheterization effectiveness: the ESCAPE trial.

Binanay C, et al. ESCAPE Investigators and ESCAPE Study Coordinators.

Journal of the American Medical Association (JAMA). 2005; October 5;294(13):1625-33.

CONTEXT:

Pulmonary artery catheters (PACs) have been used to guide therapy in multiple settings, but recent studies have raised concerns that PACs may lead to increased mortality in hospitalized patients.

OBJECTIVE:

To determine whether PAC use is safe and improves clinical outcomes in patients hospitalized with severe symptomatic and recurrent heart failure.

DESIGN, SETTING, AND PARTICIPANTS:

The Evaluation Study of Congestive Heart Failure and Pulmonary Artery Catheterization Effectiveness (ESCAPE) was a randomized controlled trial of 433 patients at 26 sites conducted from January 18, 2000, to November 17, 2003. Patients were assigned to receive therapy guided by clinical assessment and a PAC or clinical assessment alone. The target in both groups was resolution of clinical congestion, with additional PAC targets of a pulmonary capillary wedge pressure of 15 mm Hg and a right atrial pressure of 8 mm Hg. Medications were not specified, but inotrope use was explicitly discouraged.

MAIN OUTCOME MEASURES:

The primary end point was days alive out of the hospital during the first 6 months, with secondary end points of exercise, quality of life, biochemical, and echocardiographic changes.

RESULTS:

Severity of illness was reflected by the following values: average left ventricular ejection fraction, 19%; systolic blood pressure, 106 mm Hg; sodium level, 137 mEq/L; urea nitrogen, 35 mg/dL (12.40 mmol/L); and creatinine, 1.5 mg/dL (132.6 micromol/L). Therapy in both groups led to substantial reduction in symptoms, jugular venous pressure, and edema. Use of the PAC did not significantly affect the primary end point of days alive and out of the hospital during the first 6 months (133 days vs 135 days; hazard ratio [HR], 1.00 [95% confidence interval {CI}, 0.82-1.21]; P = .99), mortality (43 patients [10%] vs 38 patients [9%]; odds ratio [OR], 1.26 [95% CI, 0.78-2.03]; P = .35), or the number of days hospitalized (8.7 vs 8.3; HR, 1.04 [95% CI, 0.86-1.27]; P = .67). In-hospital adverse events were more common among patients in the PAC group (47 [21.9%] vs 25 [11.5%]; P = .04). There were no deaths related to PAC use, and no difference for in-hospital plus 30-day mortality (10 [4.7%] vs 11 [5.0%]; OR, 0.97 [95% CI, 0.38-2.22]; P = .97). Exercise and quality of life end points improved in both groups with a trend toward greater improvement with the PAC, which reached significance for the time trade-off at all time points after randomization.

CONCLUSIONS:

Therapy to reduce volume overload during hospitalization for heart failure led to marked improvement in signs and symptoms of elevated filling pressures with or without the PAC. Addition of the PAC to careful clinical assessment increased anticipated adverse events, but did not affect overall mortality and hospitalization. Future trials should test noninvasive assessments with specific treatment strategies that could be used to better tailor therapy for both survival time and survival quality as valued by patients.

REMATCH TRIAL
LONG-TERM USE OF A LEFT VENTRICULAR ASSIST DEVICE FOR END-STAGE HEART FAILURE.
NEW ENGLAND JOURNAL OF MEDICINE (NEJM). 2001.

REMATCH trial established the possibility of using mechanical support with left ventricular assist device LVAD as an alternative option for patients with advanced heart failure (in those who are not a candidate for transplant). LVAD use was associated with significant improvement in survival as well as quality of life when compared to medical therapy alone.

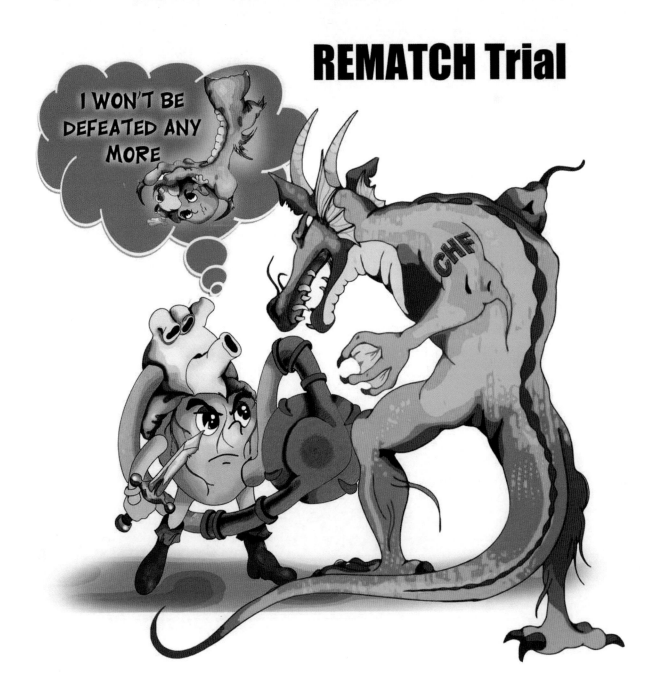

REMATCH TRIAL

Long-term use of a left ventricular assist device for end-stage heart failure.

Rose EA, et al.Randomized Evaluation of Mechanical Assistance for the Treatment of Congestive Heart Failure (REMATCH) Study Group.

New England Journal of Medicine (NEJM). 2001; November 15; 345(20):1435-43.

BACKGROUND:

Implantable left ventricular assist devices have benefited patients with end-stage heart failure as a bridge to cardiac transplantation, but their long-term use for the purpose of enhancing survival and the quality of life has not been evaluated.

METHODS:

We randomly assigned 129 patients with end-stage heart failure who were ineligible for cardiac transplantation to receive a left ventricular assist device (68 patients) or optimal medical management (61). All patients had symptoms of New York Heart Association class IV heart failure.

RESULTS:

Kaplan-Meier survival analysis showed a reduction of 48 percent in the risk of death from any cause in the group that received left ventricular assist devices as compared with the medical-therapy group (relative risk, 0.52; 95 percent confidence interval, 0.34 to 0.78; P=0.001). The rates of survival at one year were 52 percent in the device group and 25 percent in the medical-therapy group (P=0.002), and the rates at two years were 23 percent and 8 percent (P=0.09), respectively. The frequency of serious adverse events in the device group was 2.35 (95 percent confidence interval, 1.86 to 2.95) times that in the medical-therapy group, with a predominance of infection, bleeding, and malfunction of the device. The quality of life was significantly improved at one year in the device group.

CONCLUSIONS:

The use of a left ventricular assist device in patients with advanced heart failure resulted in a clinically meaningful survival benefit and an improved quality of life. A left ventricular assist device is an acceptable alternative therapy in selected patients who are not candidates for cardiac transplantation.

STITCH AND STITCH-II TRIALS

Both STITCH trials were surgical trials looking into CABG in patients with CAD. In STITCH trial CABG was compared to medical therapy alone. No significant difference in overall mortality although CABG patients had lower cardiovascular deaths. In STITCH-II trials CABG alone was compared to CABG with surgical ventricular reconstruction, to reduce the left ventricle volume, that showed no added benefit over CABG alone

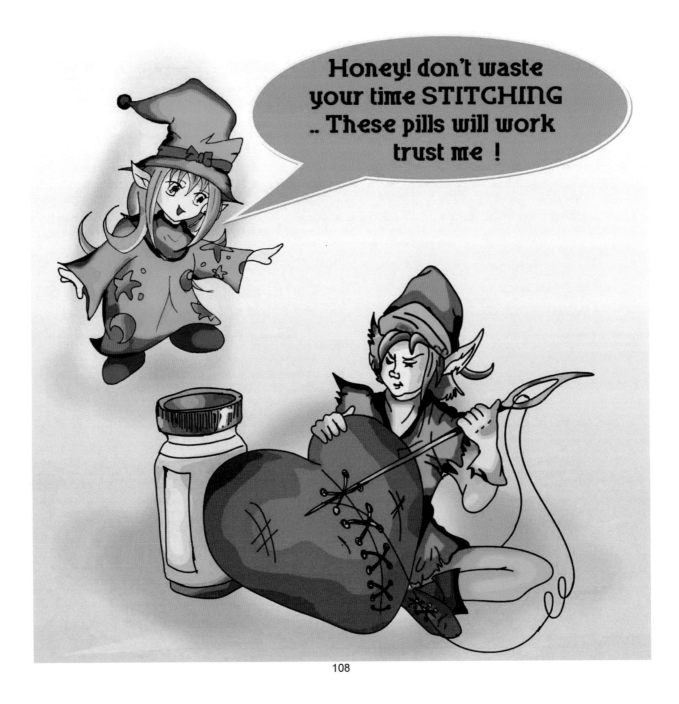

STITCH TRIAL

Coronary-artery bypass surgery in patients with left ventricular dysfunction.
Velazquez EJ, et al. STICH Investigators.
New England Journal of Medicine (NEJM). 2011; April 28; 364(17):1607-16.

BACKGROUND:

The role of coronary-artery bypass grafting (CABG) in the treatment of patients with coronary artery disease and heart failure has not been clearly established.

METHODS:

Between July 2002 and May 2007, a total of 1212 patients with an ejection fraction of 35% or less and coronary artery disease amenable to CABG were randomly assigned to medical therapy alone (602 patients) or medical therapy plus CABG (610 patients). The primary outcome was the rate of death from any cause. Major secondary outcomes included the rates of death from cardiovascular causes and of death from any cause or hospitalization for cardiovascular causes.

RESULTS:

The primary outcome occurred in 244 patients (41%) in the medical-therapy group and 218 (36%) in the CABG group (hazard ratio with CABG, 0.86; 95% confidence interval [CI], 0.72 to 1.04; P=0.12). A total of 201 patients (33%) in the medical-therapy group and 168 (28%) in the CABG group died from an adjudicated cardiovascular cause (hazard ratio with CABG, 0.81; 95% CI, 0.66 to 1.00; P=0.05). Death from any cause or hospitalization for cardiovascular causes occurred in 411 patients (68%) in the medical-therapy group and 351 (58%) in the CABG group (hazard ratio with CABG, 0.74; 95% CI, 0.64 to 0.85; P<0.001). By the end of the follo v-up period (median, 56 months), 100 patients in the medical-therapy group (17%) underwent CABG, and 555 patients in the CABG group (91%) underwent CABG.

CONCLUSIONS:

In this randomized trial, there was no significant difference between medical therapy alone and medical therapy plus CABG with respect to the primary end point of death from any cause. Patients assigned to CABG, as compared with those assigned to medical therapy alone, had lower rates of death from cardiovascular causes and of death from any cause or hospitalization for cardiovascular causes.

STITCH II TRIAL

Coronary bypass surgery with or without surgical ventricular reconstruction.
Jones RH, et al. STICH Hypothesis 2 Investigators.
New England Journal of Medicine (NEJM). 2009; April 23; 360(17):1705-17.

BACKGROUND:

Surgical ventricular reconstruction is a specific procedure designed to reduce left ventricular volume in patients with heart failure caused by coronary artery disease. We conducted a trial to address the question of whether surgical ventricular reconstruction added to coronary-artery bypass grafting (CABG) would decrease the rate of death or hospitalization for cardiac causes, as compared with CABG alone.

METHODS:

Between September 2002 and January 2006, a total of 1000 patients with an ejection fraction of 35% or less, coronary artery disease that was amenable to CABG, and dominant anterior left ventricular dysfunction that was amenable to surgical ventricular reconstruction were randomly assigned to undergo either CABG alone (499 patients) or CABG with surgical ventricular reconstruction (501 patients). The primary outcome was a composite of death from any cause and hospitalization for cardiac causes. The median follow-up was 48 months.

RESULTS:

Surgical ventricular reconstruction reduced the end-systolic volume index by 19%, as compared with a reduction of 6% with CABG alone. Cardiac symptoms and exercise tolerance improved from baseline to a similar degree in the two study groups. However, no significant difference was observed in the primary outcome, which occurred in 292 patients (59%) who were assigned to undergo CABG alone and in 289 patients (58%) who were assigned to undergo CABG with surgical ventricular reconstruction (hazard ratio for the combined approach, 0.99; 95% confidence interval, 0.84 to 1.17; P=0.90).

CONCLUSIONS:

Adding surgical ventricular reconstruction to CABG reduced the left ventricular volume, as compared with CABG alone. However, this anatomical change was not associated with a greater improvement in symptoms or exercise tolerance or with a reduction in the rate of death or hospitalization for cardiac causes.

Cardiac Electrophysiology Trials

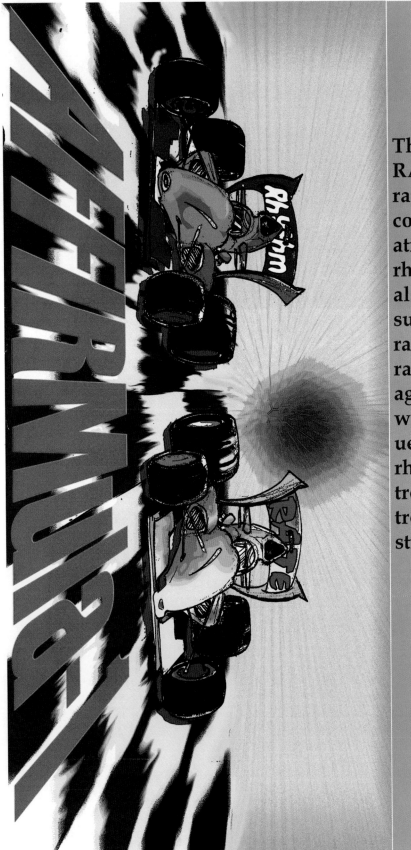

The AFFIRM and RACE trials looked into rate control vs. rhythm control in patients with atrial fibrillation. The rhythm control in both trials failed to demonstrate survival benefit, or lower rate of stroke compared to rate control with anti-coagulation. In RACE trial warfarin was discontinued after a period of sinus rhythm in the rhythm control arm, and there was trend towards increased stroke in those patients.

AFFIRM Trial
A Comparison of Rate Control and Rhythm Control in Patients with Atrial Fibrillation.
The Atrial Fibrillation Follow-up Investigation of Rhythm Management (AFFIRM)
Investigators

New England Journal of Medicine (NEJM) 2002; December 5, ; 347:1825-1833

BACKGROUND

There are two approaches to the treatment of atrial fibrillation: one is cardioversion and treatment with antiarrhythmic drugs to maintain sinus rhythm, and the other is the use of rate-controlling drugs, allowing atrial fibrillation to persist. In both approaches, the use of anticoagulant drugs is recommended.

METHODS

We conducted a randomized, multicenter comparison of these two treatment strategies in patients with atrial fibrillation and a high risk of stroke or death. The primary end point was overall mortality.

RESULTS

A total of 4060 patients (mean [±SD] age, 69.7±9.0 years) were enrolled in the study; 70.8 percent had a history of hypertension, and 38.2 percent had coronary artery disease. Of the 3311 patients with echocardiograms, the left atrium was enlarged in 64.7 percent and left ventricular function was depressed in 26.0 percent. There were 356 deaths among the patients assigned to rhythm-control therapy and 310 deaths among those assigned to rate-control therapy (mortality at five years, 23.8 percent and 21.3 percent, respectively; hazard ratio, 1.15 [95 percent confidence interval, 0.99 to 1.34]; P=0.08). More patients in the rhythm-control group than in the rate-control group were hospitalized, and there were more adverse drug effects in the rhythm-control group as well. In both groups, the majority of strokes occurred after warfarin had been stopped or when the international normalized ratio was subtherapeutic.

CONCLUSIONS

Management of atrial fibrillation with the rhythm-control strategy offers no survival advantage over the rate-control strategy, and there are potential advantages, such as a lower risk of adverse drug effects, with the rate-control strategy. Anticoagulation should be continued in this group of high-risk patients.

RACE
A comparison of rate control and rhythm control in patients with recurrent persistent atrial fibrillation.
Van Gelder IC et al , Rate Control versus Electrical Cardioversion for Persistent Atrial Fibrillation Study Group.

New England Journal of Medicine (NEJM) 2002; December 5;347(23):1834-40.

BACKGROUND:

Maintenance of sinus rhythm is the main therapeutic goal in patients with atrial fibrillation. However, recurrences of atrial fibrillation and side effects of antiarrhythmic drugs offset the benefits of sinus rhythm. We hypothesized that ventricular rate control is not inferior to the maintenance of sinus rhythm for the treatment of atrial fibrillation.

METHODS:

We randomly assigned 522 patients who had persistent atrial fibrillation after a previous electrical cardioversion to receive treatment aimed at rate control or rhythm control. Patients in the rate-control group received oral anticoagulant drugs and rate-slowing medication. Patients in the rhythm-control group underwent serial cardioversions and received antiarrhythmic drugs and oral anticoagulant drugs. The end point was a composite of death from cardiovascular causes, heart failure, thromboembolic complications, bleeding, implantation of a pacemaker, and severe adverse effects of drugs.

RESULTS:

After a mean (+/-SD) of 2.3+/-0.6 years, 39 percent of the 266 patients in the rhythm-control group had sinus rhythm, as compared with 10 percent of the 256 patients in the rate-control group. The primary end point occurred in 44 patients (17.2 percent) in the rate-control group and in 60 (22.6 percent) in the rhythm-control group. The 90 percent (two-sided) upper boundary of the absolute difference in the primary end point was 0.4 percent (the prespecified criterion for noninferiority was 10 percent or less). The distribution of the various components of the primary end point was similar in the rate-control and rhythm-control groups.

CONCLUSIONS:

Rate control is not inferior to rhythm control for the prevention of death and morbidity from cardiovascular causes and may be appropriate therapy in patients with a recurrence of persistent atrial fibrillation after electrical cardioversion.

RACE II

Lenient versus strict rate control in patients with atrial fibrillation.

Van Gelder IC, et al RACE II Investigators.

New England Journal of Medicine (NEJM) 2010; April 15;362(15):1363-73

While AFFIRM and RACE trials compared rate vs. rhythm control, RACE-II trial came to compare tight vs. loose rate control of heart rate in patients with permanent atrial fibrillation.

In that trial lenient (loose) control of the heart rate (resting heart rate is <110 bpm) was non-inferior to the strict heart rate control (resting HR was < 80 bpm); In terms of cardiovascular death, heart-failure hospitalization, stroke, and other major events.

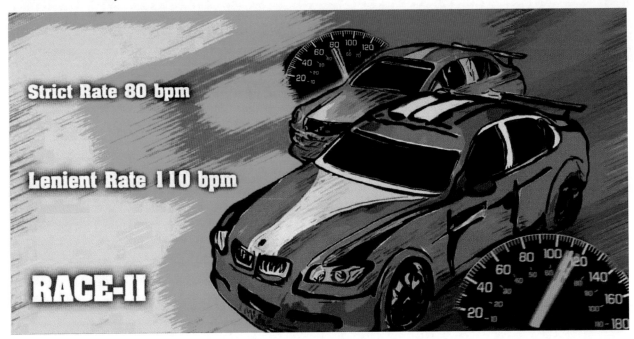

BACKGROUND:

Rate control is often the therapy of choice for atrial fibrillation. Guidelines recommend strict rate control, but this is not based on clinical evidence. We hypothesized that lenient rate control is not inferior to strict rate control for preventing cardiovascular morbidity and mortality in patients with permanent atrial fibrillation.

METHODS:

We randomly assigned 614 patients with permanent atrial fibrillation to undergo a lenient rate-control strategy (resting heart rate <110 beats per minute) or a strict rate-control strategy (resting heart rate <80 beats per minute and heart rate during moderate exercise <110 beats per minute). The primary outcome was a composite of death from cardiovascular causes, hospitalization for heart failure, and stroke, systemic embolism, bleeding, and life-threatening arrhythmic events. The duration of follow-up was at least 2 years, with a maximum of 3 years.

RESULTS:

The estimated cumulative incidence of the primary outcome at 3 years was 12.9% in the lenient-control group and 14.9% in the strict-control group, with an absolute difference with respect to the lenient-control group of -2.0 percentage points (90% confidence interval, -7.6 to 3.5; P<0.001 for the prespecified noninferiority margin). The frequencies of the components of the primary outcome were similar in the two groups. More patients in the lenient-control group met the heart-rate target or targets (304 [97.7%], vs. 203 [67.0%] in the strict-control group; P<0.001) with fewer total visits (75 [median, 0], vs. 684 [median, 2]; P<0.001). The frequencies of symptoms and adverse events were similar in the two groups.

CONCLUSIONS:

In patients with permanent atrial fibrillation, lenient rate control is as effective as strict rate control and is easier to achieve.

DIAMOND TRIALS

DIAMOND trials tested the safety and the efficacy of Dofetilide in restoring and mainataing sinus rhythm in patient with congestive heart failure (DIAMNOD-CHF), and in patients with acute MI and severe LV dysfunction (DIAMOND-MI). there was no increase in mortality with Dofetilide group vs. palcebo, and patients on Dofetilide were more likely to convert or stay in sinus rhythm. However, torsades de pointes were seen more often in patients receiving Dofetilide.

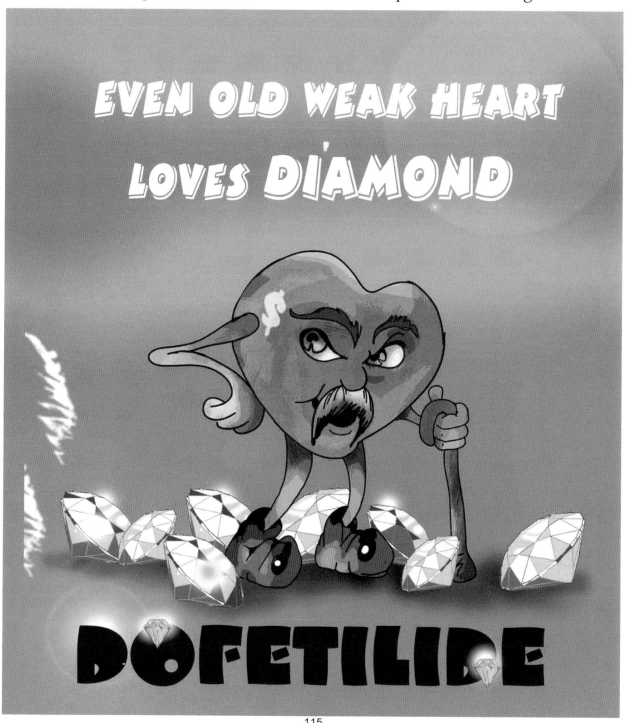

DIAMOND-CHF

Dofetilide in Patients with Congestive Heart Failure and Left Ventricular Dysfunction

Christian Torp-Pedersen et al the Danish Investigations of Arrhythmia and Mortality on Dofetilide Study Group

New England Journal of Medicine (NEJM) 1999 September 16; 341:857-865

Background

Atrial fibrillation occurs frequently in patients with congestive heart failure and commonly results in clinical deterioration and hospitalization. Sinus rhythm may be maintained with antiarrhythmic drugs, but some of these drugs increase the risk of death.

Methods

We studied 1518 patients with symptomatic congestive heart failure and severe left ventricular dysfunction at 34 Danish hospitals. We randomly assigned 762 patients to receive dofetilide, a novel class III antiarrhythmic agent, and 756 to receive placebo in a double-blind study. Treatment was initiated in the hospital and included three days of cardiac monitoring and dose adjustment. The primary end point was death from any cause.

Results

During a median follow-up of 18 months, 311 patients in the dofetilide group (41 percent) and 317 patients in the placebo group (42 percent) died (hazard ratio, 0.95; 95 percent confidence interval, 0.81 to 1.11). Treatment with dofetilide significantly reduced the risk of hospitalization for worsening congestive heart failure (risk ratio, 0.75; 95 percent confidence interval, 0.63 to 0.89). Dofetilide was effective in converting atrial fibrillation to sinus rhythm. After one month, 22 of 190 patients with atrial fibrillation at base line (12 percent) had sinus rhythm restored with dofetilide, as compared with only 3 of 201 patients (1 percent) given placebo. Once sinus rhythm was restored, dofetilide was significantly more effective than placebo in maintaining sinus rhythm (hazard ratio for the recurrence of atrial fibrillation, 0.35; 95 percent confidence interval, 0.22 to 0.57; P<0.001). There were 25 cases of torsade de pointes in the dofetilide group (3.3 percent) as compared with none in the placebo group.

Conclusions

In patients with congestive heart failure and reduced left ventricular function, dofetilide was effective in converting atrial fibrillation, preventing its recurrence, and reducing the risk of hospitalization for worsening heart failure. Dofetilide had no effect on mortality.

DIAMOND-MI

Effect of dofetilide in patients with recent myocardial infarction and left-ventricular dysfunction: a randomised trial.

Køber L, et al. Danish Investigations of Arrhythmia and Mortality on Dofetilide (DIAMOND) Study Group.

Lancet. 2000; December 16 ;356(9247):2052-8.

BACKGROUND

Arrhythmias cause much morbidity and mortality after myocardial infarction, but in previous trials, antiarrhythmic drug therapy has not been convincingly effective. Dofetilide, a new class III agent, was investigated for effects on all-cause mortality and morbidity in patients with left-ventricular dysfunction after myocardial infarction.

METHODS

In 37 Danish coronary-care units, 1510 patients with severe left-ventricular dysfunction (wall motion index < or = 1.2, corresponding to ejection fraction < or = 0.35) were enrolled in a randomised, double-blind study comparing dofetilide (n=749) with placebo (n=761). The primary endpoint was all-cause mortality. Secondary endpoints included cardiac and arrhythmic mortality and total arrhythmic deaths. Analyses were by intention to treat.

FINDINGS

No significant differences were found between the dofetilide and placebo groups in all-cause mortality (230 [31%] vs 243 [32%]), cardiac mortality (191 [26%] vs 212 [28%]), or total arrhythmic deaths (129 [17%] vs 140 [18%]). Atrial fibrillation or flutter was present in 8% of the patients at study entry. In these patients, dofetilide was significantly better than placebo at restoring sinus rhythm (25 of 59 vs seven of 56; p=0.002). There were seven cases of torsade de pointes ventricular tachycardia, all in the dofetilide group.

INTERPRETATION

In patients with severe left-ventricular dysfunction and recent myocardial infarction, treatment with dofetilide did not affect all-cause mortality, cardiac mortality, or total arrhythmic deaths. Dofetilide was effective in treating atrial fibrillation or flutter in this population.

SAFE-T
AMIODARONE VERSUS SOTALOL FOR ATRIAL FIBRILLATION.

NEW ENGLAND JOURNAL OF MEDICINE (NEJM) 2005.

SAFE-T is a Double blind clinical trial compared amiodarone, sotalol, and placebo in terms of converting patients with persistent atrial fibrillation into sinus rhythm and in maintaining sinus rhythm. No significant difference in the efficacy of converting patients into sinus rhythm between sotalol and amiodarone, while amiodarone was more potent in maintaining sinus rhythm. Both drugs were equally effective in patients with coronary artery disease.

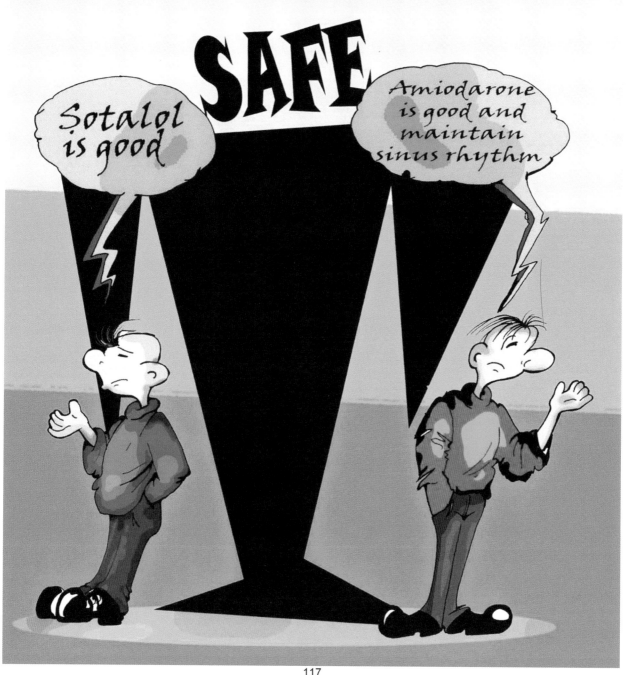

SAFE-T

Amiodarone versus sotalol for atrial fibrillation.

Singh BN, et al. Sotalol Amiodarone Atrial Fibrillation Efficacy Trial (SAFE-T) Investigators.

New England Journal of Medicine (NEJM) 2005; May 5; 352(18):1861-72.

BACKGROUND

The optimal pharmacologic means to restore and maintain sinus rhythm in patients with atrial fibrillation remains controversial.

METHODS:

In this double-blind, placebo-controlled trial, we randomly assigned 665 patients who were receiving anticoagulants and had persistent atrial fibrillation to receive amiodarone (267 patients), sotalol (261 patients), or placebo (137 patients) and monitored them for 1 to 4.5 years. The primary end point was the time to recurrence of atrial fibrillation beginning on day 28, determined by means of weekly transtelephonic monitoring.

RESULTS:

Spontaneous conversion occurred in 27.1 percent of the amiodarone group, 24.2 percent of the sotalol group, and 0.8 percent of the placebo group, and direct-current cardioversion failed in 27.7 percent, 26.5 percent, and 32.1 percent, respectively. The median times to a recurrence of atrial fibrillation were 487 days in the amiodarone group, 74 days in the sotalol group, and 6 days in the placebo group according to intention to treat and 809, 209, and 13 days, respectively, according to treatment received. Amiodarone was superior to sotalol ($P<0.001$) and to placebo ($P<0.001$), and sotalol was superior to placebo ($P<0.001$). In patients with ischemic heart disease, the median time to a recurrence of atrial fibrillation was 569 days with amiodarone therapy and 428 days with sotalol therapy ($P=0.53$). Restoration and maintenance of sinus rhythm significantly improved the quality of life and exercise capacity. There were no significant differences in major adverse events among the three groups.

CONCLUSIONS:

Amiodarone and sotalol are equally efficacious in converting atrial fibrillation to sinus rhythm. Amiodarone is superior for maintaining sinus rhythm, but both drugs have similar efficacy in patients with ischemic heart disease. Sustained sinus rhythm is associated with an improved quality of life and improved exercise performance.

MOST OF THE DRONEDARONE TRIALS WERE NAMED AFTER GREEK MYTHOLOGY

ATHENA
ANDROMEDA
EURIDIS
ADONIS
PALLAS
DIONYSOS

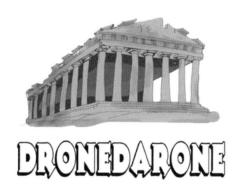

DRONEDARONE

ATHENA
EFFECT OF DRONEDARONE ON CARDIOVASCULAR EVENTS IN ATRIAL FIBRILLATION
NEW ENGLAND JOURNAL OF MEDICINE (NEJM) 2009.

Athena trial established the safety of Dronedarone in patients with atrial fibrillation / atrial flutter. Compared with placebo Dronedarone had less cardiovascular events or deaths, and showed no increase in pulmonary or thyroid toxicity. Although there was higher incidence of bradycardia, GI side effects, long QTc, and increased creatinine with the Dronedarone.

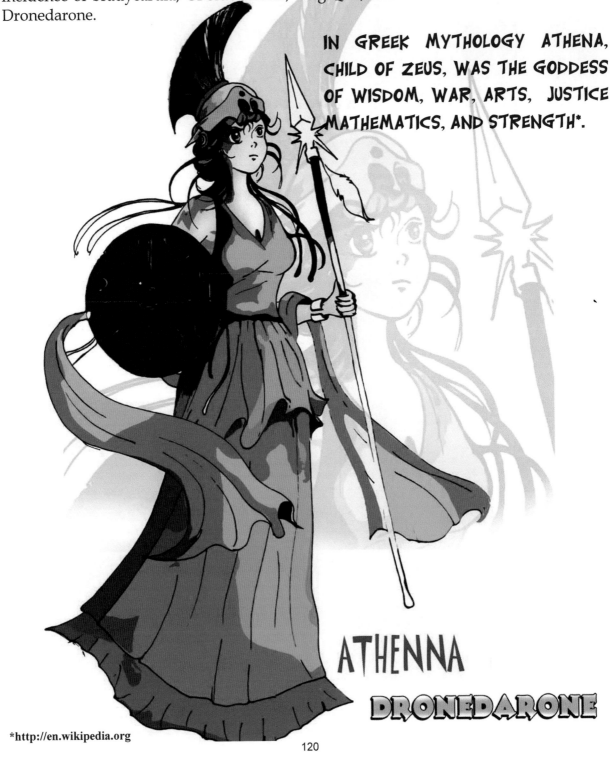

IN GREEK MYTHOLOGY ATHENA, CHILD OF ZEUS, WAS THE GODDESS OF WISDOM, WAR, ARTS, JUSTICE MATHEMATICS, AND STRENGTH*.

ATHENNA

DRONEDARONE

*http://en.wikipedia.org

ANDROMEDA

Increased Mortality after Dronedarone Therapy for Severe Heart Failure

Lars Kober et al. for the Dronedarone Study Group

New England Journal of Medicine (NEJM) 2008; June 19; 358:2678-2687

BACKGROUND

Dronedarone is a novel antiarrhythmic drug with electrophysiological properties that are similar to those of amiodarone, but it does not contain iodine and thus does not cause iodine-related adverse reactions. Therefore, it may be of value in the treatment of patients with heart failure.

METHODS

In a multicenter study with a double-blind design, we planned to randomly assign 1000 patients who were hospitalized with symptomatic heart failure and severe left ventricular systolic dysfunction to receive 400 mg of dronedarone twice a day or placebo. The primary end point was the composite of death from any cause or hospitalization for heart failure.

RESULTS

After inclusion of 627 patients (310 in the dronedarone group and 317 in the placebo group), the trial was prematurely terminated for safety reasons, at the recommendation of the data and safety monitoring board, in accordance with the board's predefined rules for termination of the study. During a median follow-up of 2 months, 25 patients in the dronedarone group (8.1%) and 12 patients in the placebo group (3.8%) died (hazard ratio in the dronedarone group, 2.13; 95% confidence interval [CI], 1.07 to 4.25; P=0.03). The excess mortality was predominantly related to worsening of heart failure — 10 deaths in the dronedarone group and 2 in the placebo group. The primary end point did not differ significantly between the two groups; there were 53 events in the dronedarone group (17.1%) and 40 events in the placebo group (12.6%) (hazard ratio, 1.38; 95% CI, 0.92 to 2.09; P=0.12). More increases in the creatinine concentration were reported as serious adverse events in the dronedarone group than in the placebo group.

CONCLUSIONS

In patients with severe heart failure and left ventricular systolic dysfunction, treatment with dronedarone was associated with increased early mortality related to the worsening of heart failure.

ANDROMEDA

INCREASED MORTALITY AFTER DRONEDARONE THERAPY FOR SEVERE HEART FAILURE
LARS KOBER ET AL. FOR THE DRONEDARONE STUDY GROUP
NEW ENGLAND JOURNAL OF MEDICINE (NEJM) 2008

Dronedarone is a novel multichannel blocker with electrophysiological properties similar to those of amiodarone. Andromeda trial was designed to test the hypothesis that Dronedarone would reduce the rate of hospitalization due to heart failure and possibly reduce mortality caused by arrhythmia. However, Dronedarone doubled the mortality in patients with LV dysfunction and Andromeda trial was terminated early. Mortalities were related to the worsening of heart failure.

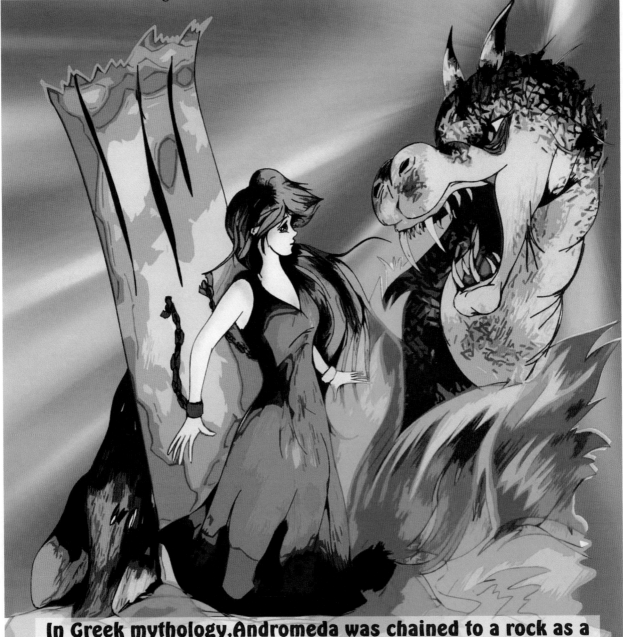

In Greek mythology, Andromeda was chained to a rock as a sacrifice to sea monster, but she was saved by Perseus*.

*http://en.wikipedia.org

ANDROMEDA

Increased Mortality after Dronedarone Therapy for Severe Heart Failure

Lars Kober et al. for the Dronedarone Study Group

New England Journal of Medicine (NEJM) 2008; June 19; 358:2678-2687.

BACKGROUND

Dronedarone is a novel antiarrhythmic drug with electrophysiological properties that are similar to those of amiodarone, but it does not contain iodine and thus does not cause iodine-related adverse reactions. Therefore, it may be of value in the treatment of patients with heart failure.

METHODS

In a multicenter study with a double-blind design, we planned to randomly assign 1000 patients who were hospitalized with symptomatic heart failure and severe left ventricular systolic dysfunction to receive 400 mg of dronedarone twice a day or placebo. The primary end point was the composite of death from any cause or hospitalization for heart failure.

RESULTS

After inclusion of 627 patients (310 in the dronedarone group and 317 in the placebo group), the trial was prematurely terminated for safety reasons, at the recommendation of the data and safety monitoring board, in accordance with the board's predefined rules for termination of the study. During a median follow-up of 2 months, 25 patients in the dronedarone group (8.1%) and 12 patients in the placebo group (3.8%) died (hazard ratio in the dronedarone group, 2.13; 95% confidence interval [CI], 1.07 to 4.25; P=0.03). The excess mortality was predominantly related to worsening of heart failure — 10 deaths in the dronedarone group and 2 in the placebo group. The primary end point did not differ significantly between the two groups; there were 53 events in the dronedarone group (17.1%) and 40 events in the placebo group (12.6%) (hazard ratio, 1.38; 95% CI, 0.92 to 2.09; P=0.12). More increases in the creatinine concentration were reported as serious adverse events in the dronedarone group than in the placebo group.

CONCLUSIONS

In patients with severe heart failure and left ventricular systolic dysfunction, treatment with dronedarone was associated with increased early mortality related to the worsening of heart failure.

EURIDIS AND ADONIS TRIALS

DRONEDARONE FOR MAINTENANCE OF SINUS RHYTHM IN ATRIAL FIBRILLATION OR FLUTTER.
NEW ENGLAND JOURNAL OF MEDICINE (NEJM) 2007.

These two trials compared Dronedarone to placebo in patients with atrial fibrillation and atrial flutter, and both demonstrated that Dronedarone was more effective than placebo in maintaining sinus rhythm and in reducing the ventricular rate during recurrence of arrhythmia.

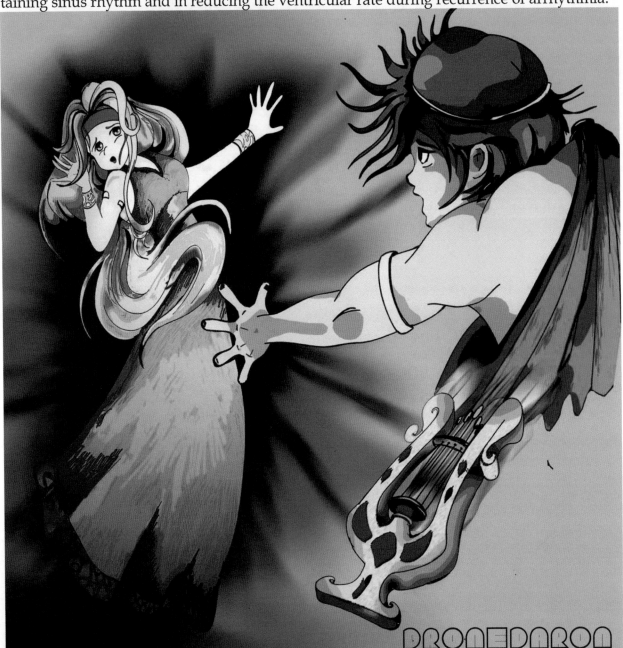

Eurydice was the beautiful wife of Orpheus, she died after a snake bite. Her grieving husband went to the underworld where he was able to soften the heart of Hades (the Greek god of the underworld) with his enchanting music. Hades allowed Orpheus to take his wife back with one condition, he can't look at her until they reach the upper-world. Orpheus walked in front of her and few steps before he reaches the upper-world, he could not resist and he looked back, and Eurydice vanished into the darkness of the underworld again*.

*http://en.wikipedia.org

EURIDIS and ADONIS Trials

Dronedarone for maintenance of sinus rhythm in atrial fibrillation or flutter.

Singh BN, et al. EURIDIS and ADONIS Investigators.

New England Journal of Medicine (NEJM) 2007; September 6; 357(10):987-99.

BACKGROUND

Amiodarone is effective in maintaining sinus rhythm in atrial fibrillation but is associated with potentially serious toxic effects. Dronedarone is a new antiarrhythmic agent pharmacologically related to amiodarone but developed to reduce the risk of side effects.

METHODS

In two identical multicenter, double-blind, randomized trials, one conducted in Europe (ClinicalTrials.gov number, NCT00259428 [ClinicalTrials.gov]) and one conducted in the United States, Canada, Australia, South Africa, and Argentina (termed the non-European trial, NCT00259376 [ClinicalTrials.gov]), we evaluated the efficacy of dronedarone, with 828 patients receiving 400 mg of the drug twice daily and 409 patients receiving placebo. Rhythm was monitored transtelephonically on days 2, 3, and 5; at 3, 5, 7, and 10 months; during recurrence of arrhythmia; and at nine scheduled visits during a 12-month period. The primary end point was the time to the first recurrence of atrial fibrillation or flutter.

RESULTS

In the European trial, the median times to the recurrence of arrhythmia were 41 days in the placebo group and 96 days in the dronedarone group (P=0.01). The corresponding durations in the non-European trial were 59 and 158 days (P=0.002). At the recurrence of arrhythmia in the European trial, the mean (+/-SD) ventricular rate was 117.5+/-29.1 beats per minute in the placebo group and 102.3+/-24.7 beats per minute in the dronedarone group (P<0.001); the corresponding rates in the non-European trial were 116.6+/-31.9 and 104.6+/-27.1 beats per minute (P<0.001). Rates of pulmonary toxic effects and of thyroid and liver dysfunction were not significantly increased in the dronedarone group.

CONCLUSIONS

Dronedarone was significantly more effective than placebo in maintaining sinus rhythm and in reducing the ventricular rate during recurrence of arrhythmia.

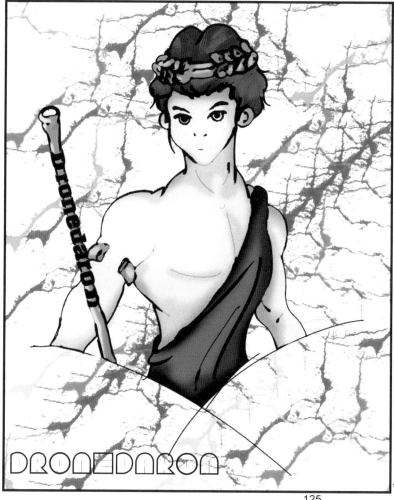

Adonis, in Greek mythology, is the demigod of beauty and desire*.

*http://en.wikipedia.org

PALLAS TRIAL
DRONEDARONE IN HIGH-RISK PERMANENT ATRIAL FIBRILLATION
NEW ENGLAND JOURNAL OF MEDICINE (NEJM) 2011.

All previous Dronedarone trials tested the drug in intermittent atrial fibrillation or atrial flutter, PALLAS trials hypnotized that similar benefit can be seen in patients with permanent atrial fibrillation. However, the results came out contrary to the hypothesis and Dronedarone actually increased the cardiovascular events in these patients.

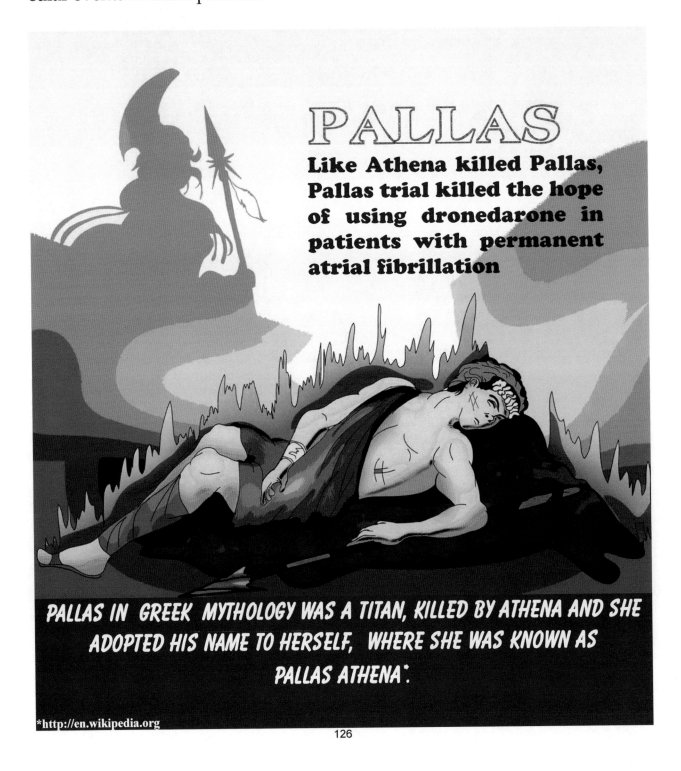

PALLAS

Like Athena killed Pallas, Pallas trial killed the hope of using dronedarone in patients with permanent atrial fibrillation

PALLAS IN GREEK MYTHOLOGY WAS A TITAN, KILLED BY ATHENA AND SHE ADOPTED HIS NAME TO HERSELF, WHERE SHE WAS KNOWN AS PALLAS ATHENA*.

*http://en.wikipedia.org

PALLAS TRIAL

Dronedarone in High-Risk Permanent Atrial Fibrillation

Stuart J. Connolly, M.D et al.

New England Journal of Medicine (NEJM). 2011; December 15; 365:2268-2276 .

BACKGROUND:

Dronedarone restores sinus rhythm and reduces hospitalization or death in intermittent atrial fibrillation. It also lowers heart rate and blood pressure and has antiadrenergic and potential ventricular antiarrhythmic effects. We hypothesized that dronedarone would reduce major vascular events in high-risk permanent atrial fibrillation.

METHODS:

We assigned patients who were at least 65 years of age with at least a 6-month history of permanent atrial fibrillation and risk factors for major vascular events to receive dronedarone or placebo. The first coprimary outcome was stroke, myocardial infarction, systemic embolism, or death from cardiovascular causes. The second coprimary outcome was unplanned hospitalization for a cardiovascular cause or death.

RESULTS:

After the enrollment of 3236 patients, the study was stopped for safety reasons. The first coprimary outcome occurred in 43 patients receiving dronedarone and 19 receiving placebo (hazard ratio, 2.29; 95% confidence interval [CI], 1.34 to 3.94; P=0.002). There were 21 deaths from cardiovascular causes in the dronedarone group and 10 in the placebo group (hazard ratio, 2.11; 95% CI, 1.00 to 4.49; P=0.046), including death from arrhythmia in 13 patients and 4 patients, respectively (hazard ratio, 3.26; 95% CI, 1.06 to 10.00; P=0.03). Stroke occurred in 23 patients in the dronedarone group and 10 in the placebo group (hazard ratio, 2.32; 95% CI, 1.11 to 4.88; P=0.02). Hospitalization for heart failure occurred in 43 patients in the dronedarone group and 24 in the placebo group (hazard ratio, 1.81; 95% CI, 1.10 to 2.99; P=0.02).

CONCLUSIONS:

Dronedarone increased rates of heart failure, stroke, and death from cardiovascular causes in patients with permanent atrial fibrillation who were at risk for major vascular events. Our data show that this drug should not be used in such patients.

DIONYSOS

A SHORT-TERM, RANDOMIZED, DOUBLE-BLIND, PARALLEL-GROUP STUDY TO EVALUATE THE EFFICACY AND SAFETY OF DRONEDARONE VERSUS AMIODARONE IN PATIENTS WITH PERSISTENT ATRIAL FIBRILLATION: THE DIONYSOS STUDY.

JOURNAL OF CARDIOVASCULAR ELECTROPHYSIOLOGY (JCE) 2010

DIONYSOS trial compared amiodarone to Dronedarone in patients with persistent atrial fibrillation. Dronedarone was found to be less effective in decreasing AF recurrence, but had a better safety profile, specifically with regard to thyroid and neurologic events and a lack of interaction with oral anticoagulants.

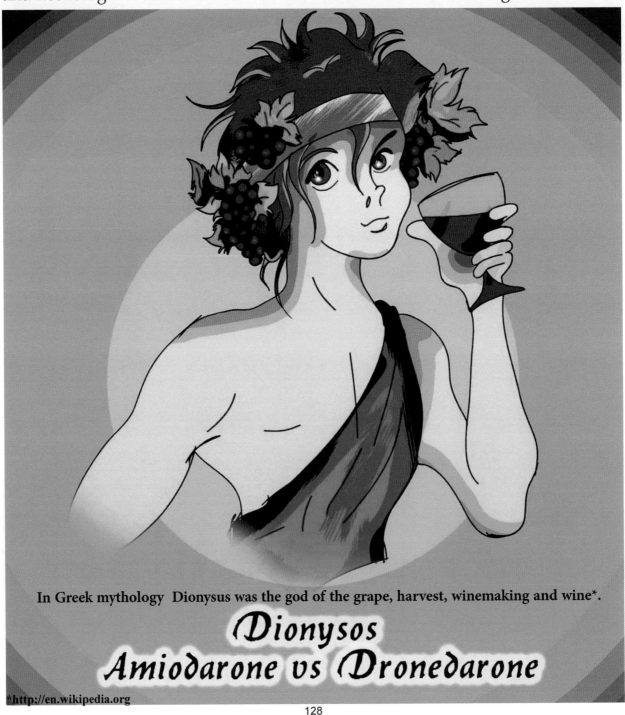

In Greek mythology Dionysus was the god of the grape, harvest, winemaking and wine*.

Dionysos
Amiodarone vs Dronedarone

*http://en.wikipedia.org

DIONYSOS

A short-term, randomized, double-blind, parallel-group study to evaluate the efficacy and safety of dronedarone versus amiodarone in patients with persistent atrial fibrillation: the DIONYSOS study.

Le Heuzey JY, et al

Journal of cardiovascular electrophysiology (JCE) 2010; June 1;21(6):597-605.

INTRODUCTION:

We compared the efficacy and safety of amiodarone and dronedarone in patients with persistent atrial fibrillation (AF).

METHODS:

Five hundred and four amiodarone-naïve patients were randomized to receive dronedarone 400 mg bid (n = 249) or amiodarone 600 mg qd for 28 days then 200 mg qd (n = 255) for at least 6 months. Primary composite endpoint was recurrence of AF (including unsuccessful electrical cardioversion, no spontaneous conversion and no electrical cardioversion) or premature study discontinuation. Main safety endpoint (MSE) was occurrence of thyroid-, hepatic-, pulmonary-, neurologic-, skin-, eye-, or gastrointestinal-specific events, or premature study drug discontinuation following an adverse event.

RESULTS:

Median treatment duration was 7 months. The primary composite endpoint was 75.1 and 58.8% with dronedarone and amiodarone, respectively, at 12 months (hazard ratio [HR] 1.59; 95% confidence interval [CI] 1.28-1.98; $P < 0.0001$), mainly driven by AF recurrence with dronedarone compared with amiodarone (63.5 vs 42.0%). AF recurrence after successful cardioversion was 36.5 and 24.3% with dronedarone and amiodarone, respectively. Premature drug discontinuation tended to be less frequent with dronedarone (10.4 vs 13.3%). MSE was 39.3 and 44.5% with dronedarone and amiodarone, respectively, at 12 months (HR = 0.80; 95% CI 0.60-1.07; $P = 0.129$), and mainly driven by fewer thyroid, neurologic, skin, and ocular events in the dronedarone group.

CONCLUSION:

In this short-term study, dronedarone was less effective than amiodarone in decreasing AF recurrence, but had a better safety profile, specifically with regard to thyroid and neurologic events and a lack of interaction with oral anticoagulants.

RELY TRIAL

DABIGATRAN VERSUS WARFARIN IN PATIENTS WITH ATRIAL FIBRILLATION.
NEW ENGLAND JOURNAL OF MEDICINE (NEJM) 2009.

Dabigatran (Pradaxa) is a novel oral anticoagulant from the class of the direct thrombin inhibitors. It was compared in RELY trial to warfarin, two doses were given during the trial, the 110 mg bid was similar to warfarin in terms of strokes, while the 150 mg bid were associated with lower rate of stroke than warfarin with similar rate of major hemorrhage.

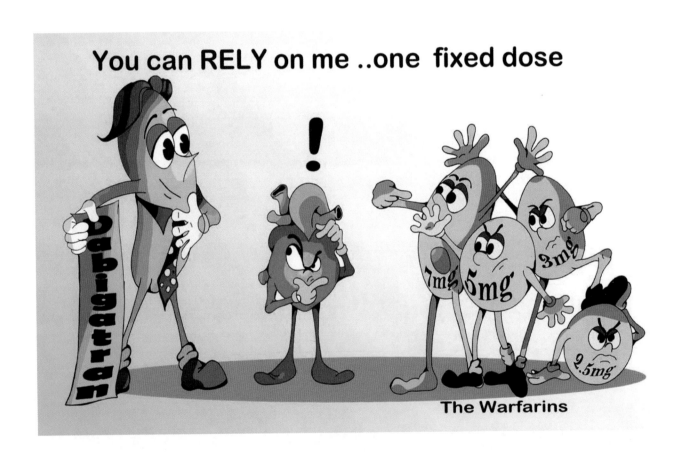

RELY Trial

Dabigatran versus warfarin in patients with atrial fibrillation.
Connolly SJ, et al. RE-LY Steering Committee and Investigators.

The New England Journal of Medicine (NEJM) 2009 September 17; 361(12):1139-51.

BACKGROUND:

Warfarin reduces the risk of stroke in patients with atrial fibrillation but increases the risk of hemorrhage and is difficult to use. Dabigatran is a new oral direct thrombin inhibitor.

METHODS:

In this non-inferiority trial, we randomly assigned 18,113 patients who had atrial fibrillation and a risk of stroke to receive, in a blinded fashion, fixed doses of dabigatran--110 mg or 150 mg twice daily--or, in an unblinded fashion, adjusted-dose warfarin. The median duration of the follow-up period was 2.0 years. The primary outcome was stroke or systemic embolism.

RESULTS:

Rates of the primary outcome were 1.69% per year in the warfarin group, as compared with 1.53% per year in the group that received 110 mg of dabigatran (relative risk with dabigatran, 0.91; 95% confidence interval [CI], 0.74 to 1.11; $P<0.001$ for noninferiority) and 1.11% per year in the group that received 150 mg of dabigatran (relative risk, 0.66; 95% CI, 0.53 to 0.82; $P<0.001$ for superiority). The rate of major bleeding was 3.36% per year in the warfarin group, as compared with 2.71% per year in the group receiving 110 mg of dabigatran ($P=0.003$) and 3.11% per year in the group receiving 150 mg of dabigatran ($P=0.31$). The rate of hemorrhagic stroke was 0.38% per year in the warfarin group, as compared with 0.12% per year with 110 mg of dabigatran ($P<0.001$) and 0.10% per year with 150 mg of dabigatran ($P<0.001$). The mortality rate was 4.13% per year in the warfarin group, as compared with 3.75% per year with 110 mg of dabigatran ($P=0.13$) and 3.64% per year with 150 mg of dabigatran ($P=0.051$).

CONCLUSIONS:

In patients with atrial fibrillation, dabigatran given at a dose of 110 mg was associated with rates of stroke and systemic embolism that were similar to those associated with warfarin, as well as lower rates of major hemorrhage. Dabigatran administered at a dose of 150 mg, as compared with warfarin, was associated with lower rates of stroke and systemic embolism but similar rates of major hemorrhage.

ROCKET AF
RIVAROXABAN VERSUS WARFARIN IN NONVALVULAR ATRIAL FIBRILLATION.
NEW ENGLAND JOURNAL OF MEDICINE (NEJM) 2011.

Rivaroxaban (Xarelto) is a new oral factor Xa inhibitor, ROCKET AF Trial compared rivaroxaban to warfarin in preventing strokes in moderate- or high-risk patients with atrial fibrillation. Rivaroxaban was proven to be non-inferior to warfarin without an increase in major bleeding.

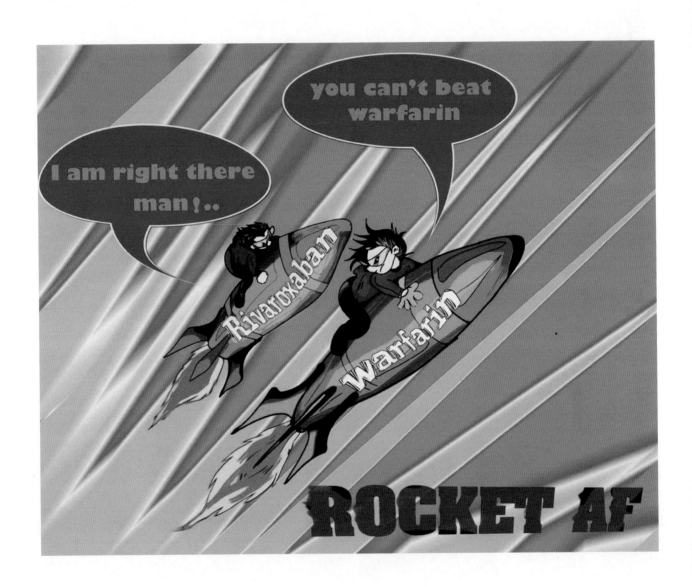

ROCKET AF

Rivaroxaban versus warfarin in nonvalvular atrial fibrillation.
Patel MR, et al. ROCKET AF Investigators.

New England Journal of Medicine (NEJM) 2011; September 8; 365(10):883-91

BACKGROUND

The use of warfarin reduces the rate of ischemic stroke in patients with atrial fibrillation but requires frequent monitoring and dose adjustment. Rivaroxaban, an oral factor Xa inhibitor, may provide more consistent and predictable anticoagulation than warfarin.

METHODS

In a double-blind trial, we randomly assigned 14,264 patients with nonvalvular atrial fibrillation who were at increased risk for stroke to receive either rivaroxaban (at a daily dose of 20 mg) or dose-adjusted warfarin. The per-protocol, as-treated primary analysis was designed to determine whether rivaroxaban was noninferior to warfarin for the primary end point of stroke or systemic embolism.

RESULTS

In the primary analysis, the primary end point occurred in 188 patients in the rivaroxaban group (1.7% per year) and in 241 in the warfarin group (2.2% per year) (hazard ratio in the rivaroxaban group, 0.79; 95% confidence interval [CI], 0.66 to 0.96; $P<0.001$ for noninferiority). In the intention-to-treat analysis, the primary end point occurred in 269 patients in the rivaroxaban group (2.1% per year) and in 306 patients in the warfarin group (2.4% per year) (hazard ratio, 0.88; 95% CI, 0.74 to 1.03; $P<0.001$ for noninferiority; $P=0.12$ for superiority). Major and nonmajor clinically relevant bleeding occurred in 1475 patients in the rivaroxaban group (14.9% per year) and in 1449 in the warfarin group (14.5% per year) (hazard ratio, 1.03; 95% CI, 0.96 to 1.11; $P=0.44$), with significant reductions in intracranial hemorrhage (0.5% vs. 0.7%, $P=0.02$) and fatal bleeding (0.2% vs. 0.5%, $P=0.003$) in the rivaroxaban group.

CONCLUSIONS

In patients with atrial fibrillation, rivaroxaban was noninferior to warfarin for the prevention of stroke or systemic embolism. There was no significant between-group difference in the risk of major bleeding, although intracranial and fatal bleeding occurred less frequently in the rivaroxaban group.

ARISTOTLE TRIAL

APIXABAN VERSUS WARFARIN IN PATIENTS WITH ATRIAL FIBRILLATION.

NEW ENGLAND JOURNAL OF MEDICINE (NEJM). 2011.

Apixaban is another factor Xa inhibitor that was proven to be effective as a strategy for anticoagulation in the management of non-valvular atrial fibrillation. While in Rocket-AF Rivaroxaban was just non-inferior (probably in a higher risk population than those included in ARISTOTLE), Apixaban was superior to warfarin not only in preventing stroke or systemic embolism, but also in cutting the rates of all complications including both bleeding, and mortality.

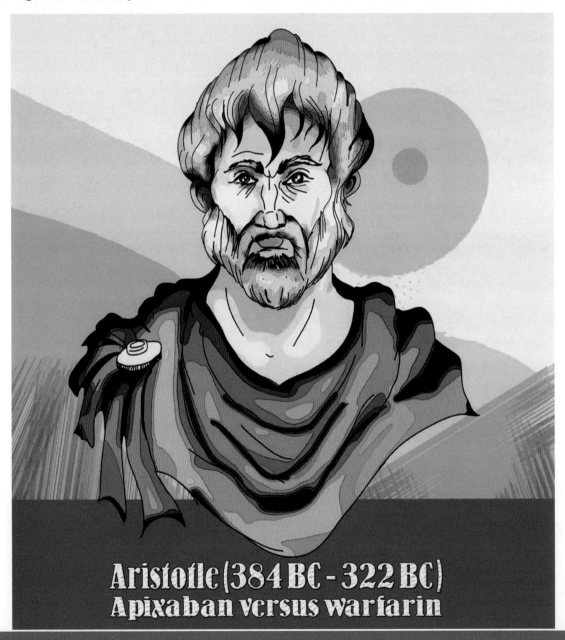

Aristotle (384 BC - 322 BC)
Apixaban versus warfarin

Aristotle was one of the greatest Greek philosophers and polymath. He was student of Plato and teacher of Alexander the Great.

*http://en.wikipedia.org

134

ARISTOTLE TRIAL

Apixaban versus warfarin in patients with atrial fibrillation.
Granger CB, et al. ARISTOTLE Committees and Investigators.

New England Journal of Medicine (NEJM). 2011; September 15; 365(11):981-92.

BACKGROUND:

Vitamin K antagonists are highly effective in preventing stroke in patients with atrial fibrillation but have several limitations. Apixaban is a novel oral direct factor Xa inhibitor that has been shown to reduce the risk of stroke in a similar population in comparison with aspirin.

METHODS:

In this randomized, double-blind trial, we compared apixaban (at a dose of 5 mg twice daily) with warfarin (target international normalized ratio, 2.0 to 3.0) in 18,201 patients with atrial fibrillation and at least one additional risk factor for stroke. The primary outcome was ischemic or hemorrhagic stroke or systemic embolism. The trial was designed to test for noninferiority, with key secondary objectives of testing for superiority with respect to the primary outcome and to the rates of major bleeding and death from any cause.

RESULTS:

The median duration of follow-up was 1.8 years. The rate of the primary outcome was 1.27% per year in the apixaban group, as compared with 1.60% per year in the warfarin group (hazard ratio with apixaban, 0.79; 95% confidence interval [CI], 0.66 to 0.95; P<0.001 for noninferiority; P=0.01 for superiority). The rate of major bleeding was 2.13% per year in the apixaban group, as compared with 3.09% per year in the warfarin group (hazard ratio, 0.69; 95% CI, 0.60 to 0.80; P<0.001), and the rates of death from any cause were 3.52% and 3.94%, respectively (hazard ratio, 0.89; 95% CI, 0.80 to 0.99; P=0.047). The rate of hemorrhagic stroke was 0.24% per year in the apixaban group, as compared with 0.47% per year in the warfarin group (hazard ratio, 0.51; 95% CI, 0.35 to 0.75; P<0.001), and the rate of ischemic or uncertain type of stroke was 0.97% per year in the apixaban group and 1.05% per year in the warfarin group (hazard ratio, 0.92; 95% CI, 0.74 to 1.13; P=0.42).

CONCLUSIONS:

In patients with atrial fibrillation, apixaban was superior to warfarin in preventing stroke or systemic embolism, caused less bleeding, and resulted in lower mortality.

APAF STUDY

A RANDOMIZED TRIAL OF CIRCUMFERENTIAL PULMONARY VEIN ABLATION VERSUS ANTIAR-RHYTHMIC DRUG THERAPY IN PAROXYSMAL ATRIAL FIBRILLATION: THE APAF STUDY.
JOURNAL OF THE AMERICAN COLLEGE OF CARDIOLOGY (JACC) 2006.

In APAF trial patients with paroxysmal atrial fibrillation who failed treatment with anti-arrhythmic drugs were randomized to circumferential pulmonary vein isolation vs. maximum dose of different anti-arrhythmic drug. The ablation group were more likely to be free of atrial fibrillation.

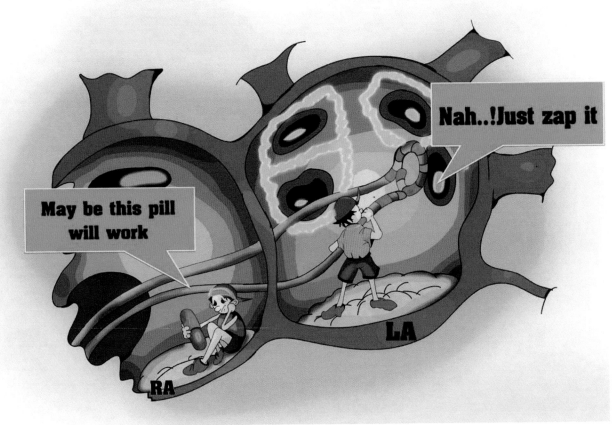

APAF Study

A randomized trial of circumferential pulmonary vein ablation versus antiarrhythmic drug therapy in paroxysmal atrial fibrillation: the APAF Study.

Pappone C et al.

Journal of the American College of Cardiology (JACC) 2006; December 5; 48(11):2340-7.

OBJECTIVES

We compared ablation strategy with antiarrhythmic drug therapy (ADT) in patients with paroxysmal atrial fibrillation (PAF).

BACKGROUND

Atrial fibrillation (AF) ablation strategy is superior to ADT in patients with an initial history of PAF, but its role in patients with a long history of AF as compared with ADT remains a challenge.

METHODS

One hundred ninety-eight patients (age, 56 +/- 10 years) with PAF of 6 +/- 5 years' duration (mean AF episodes 3.4/month) who had failed ADT were randomized to AF ablation by circumferential pulmonary vein ablation (CPVA) or to the maximum tolerable doses of another ADT, which included flecainide, sotalol, and amiodarone. Crossover to CPVA was allowed after 3 months of ADT.

RESULTS

By Kaplan-Meier analysis, 86% of patients in the CPVA group and 22% of those in the ADT group who did not require a second ADT were free from recurrent atrial tachyarrhythmias (AT) (p < 0.001); a repeat ablation was performed in 9% of patients in the CPVA group for recurrent AF (6%) or atrial tachycardia (3%). At 1 year, 93% and 35% of the CPVA and ADT groups, respectively, were AT-free. Ejection fraction, hypertension, and age independently predicted AF recurrences in the ADT group. Circumferential pulmonary vein ablation was associated with fewer cardiovascular hospitalizations (p < 0.01). One transient ischemic attack and 1 pericardial effusion occurred in the CPVA group; side effects of ADT were observed in 23 patients.

CONCLUSIONS

Circumferential pulmonary vein ablation is more successful than ADT for prevention of PAF with few complications. Atrial fibrillation ablation warrants consideration in selected patients in whom ADT had already failed and maintenance of sinus rhythm is desired.

STOP-AF TRIAL

CRYOBALLOON ABLATION OF PULMONARY VEINS FOR PAROXYSMAL ATRIAL FIBRILLATION: FIRST RESULTS OF THE NORTH AMERICAN ARCTIC FRONT (STOP AF) PIVOTAL TRIAL.
JOURNAL OF THE AMERICAN COLLEGE OF CARDIOLOGY (JACC) 2013.

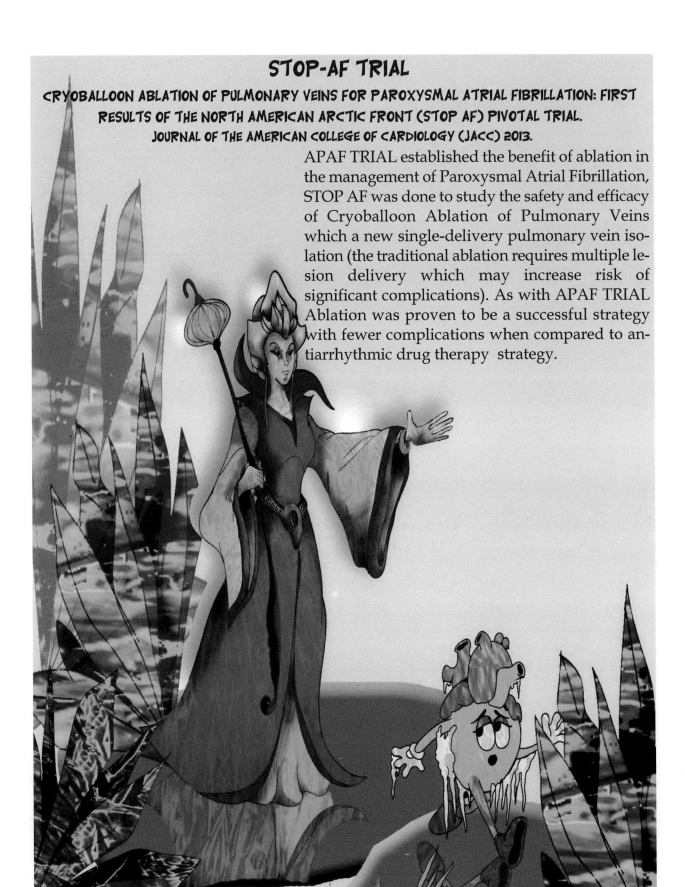

APAF TRIAL established the benefit of ablation in the management of Paroxysmal Atrial Fibrillation, STOP AF was done to study the safety and efficacy of Cryoballoon Ablation of Pulmonary Veins which a new single-delivery pulmonary vein isolation (the traditional ablation requires multiple lesion delivery which may increase risk of significant complications). As with APAF TRIAL Ablation was proven to be a successful strategy with fewer complications when compared to antiarrhythmic drug therapy strategy.

STOP-AF Trial

Cryoballoon Ablation of Pulmonary Veins for Paroxysmal Atrial Fibrillation: First Results of the North American Arctic Front (STOP AF) Pivotal Trial.

Packer DL, et al. STOP AF Cryoablation Investigators.

Journal of the American College of Cardiology (JACC) 2013; April 23; 61(16):1713-23.

OBJECTIVES:

This study sought to assess the safety and effectiveness of a novel cryoballoon ablation technology designed to achieve single-delivery pulmonary vein (PV) isolation.

BACKGROUND:

Standard radiofrequency ablation is effective in eliminating atrial fibrillation (AF) but requires multiple lesion delivery at the risk of significant complications.

METHODS:

Patients with documented symptomatic paroxysmal AF and previously failed therapy with ≥1 membrane active antiarrhythmic drug underwent 2:1 randomization to either cryoballoon ablation (n = 163) or drug therapy (n = 82). A 90-day blanking period allowed for optimization of antiarrhythmic drug therapy and reablation if necessary. Effectiveness of the cryoablation procedure versus drug therapy was determined at 12 months.

RESULTS:

Patients had highly symptomatic AF (78% paroxysmal, 22% early persistent) and experienced failure of at least one antiarrhythmic drug. Cryoablation produced acute isolation of three or more PVs in 98.2% and all four PVs in 97.6% of patients. PVs isolation was achieved with the balloon catheter alone in 83%. At 12 months, treatment success was 69.9% (114 of 163) of cryoblation patients compared with 7.3% of antiarrhythmic drug patients (absolute difference, 62.6% [p < 0.001]). Sixty-five (79%) drug-treated patients crossed over to cryoablation during 12 months of study follow-up due to recurrent, symptomatic AF, constituting drug treatment failure. There were 7 of the resulting 228 cryoablated patients (3.1%) with a >75% reduction in PV area during 12 months of follow-up. Twenty-nine of 259 procedures (11.2%) were associated with phrenic nerve palsy as determined by radiographic screening; 25 of these had resolved by 12 months. Cryoablation patients had significantly improved symptoms at 12 months.

CONCLUSIONS:

The STOP AF trial demonstrated that cryoballoon ablation is a safe and effective alternative to antiarrhythmic medication for the treatment of patients with symptomatic paroxysmal AF, for whom at least one antiarrhythmic drug has failed, with risks within accepted standards for ablation therapy.

CAST TRIAL

PRELIMINARY REPORT: EFFECT OF ENCAINIDE AND FLECAINIDE ON MORTALITY IN A RANDOMIZED TRIAL OF ARRHYTHMIA SUPPRESSION AFTER MYOCARDIAL INFARCTION.
NEW ENGLAND JOURNAL OF MEDICINE (NEJM) 1989

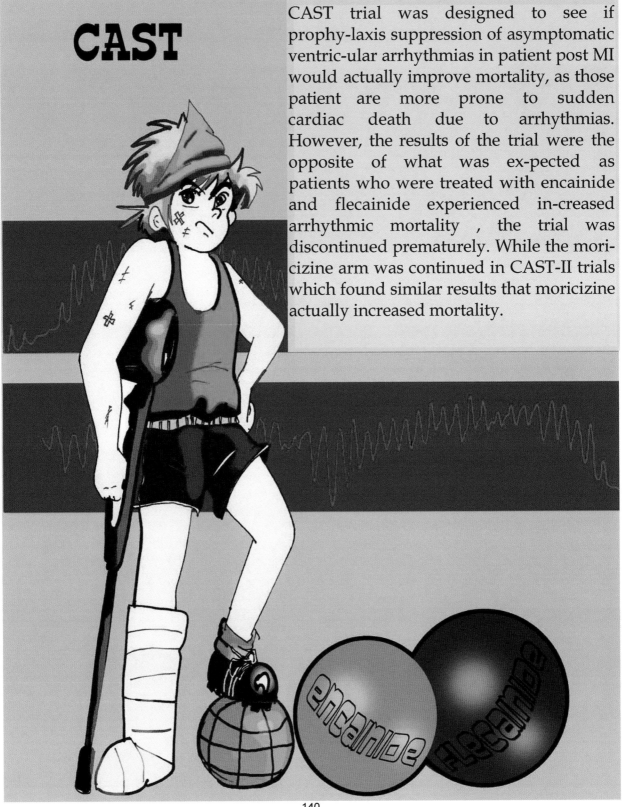

CAST trial was designed to see if prophy-laxis suppression of asymptomatic ventric-ular arrhythmias in patient post MI would actually improve mortality, as those patient are more prone to sudden cardiac death due to arrhythmias. However, the results of the trial were the opposite of what was ex-pected as patients who were treated with encainide and flecainide experienced in-creased arrhythmic mortality , the trial was discontinued prematurely. While the mori-cizine arm was continued in CAST-II trials which found similar results that moricizine actually increased mortality.

CAST Trial

Preliminary report: effect of encainide and flecainide on mortality in a randomized trial of arrhythmia suppression after myocardial infarction. The Cardiac Arrhythmia Suppression Trial (CAST) Investigators.

New England Journal of Medicine (NEJM) 1989; August 10; 321(6):406-12

The occurrence of ventricular premature depolarizations in survivors of myocardial infarction is a risk factor for subsequent sudden death, but whether antiarrhythmic therapy reduces the risk is not known. The Cardiac Arrhythmia Suppression Trial (CAST) is evaluating the effect of antiarrhythmic therapy (encainide, flecainide, or moricizine) in patients with asymptomatic or mildly symptomatic ventricular arrhythmia (six or more ventricular premature beats per hour) after myocardial infarction. As of March 30, 1989, 2309 patients had been recruited for the initial drug-titration phase of the study: 1727 (75 percent) had initial suppression of their arrhythmia (as assessed by Holter recording) through the use of one of the three study drugs and had been randomly assigned to receive active drug or placebo. During an average of 10 months of follow-up, the patients treated with active drug had a higher rate of death from arrhythmia than the patients assigned to placebo. Encainide and flecainide accounted for the excess of deaths from arrhythmia and nonfatal cardiac arrests (33 of 730 patients taking encainide or flecainide [4.5 percent]; 9 of 725 taking placebo [1.2 percent]; relative risk, 3.6; 95 percent confidence interval, 1.7 to 8.5). They also accounted for the higher total mortality (56 of 730 [7.7 percent] and 22 of 725 [3.0 percent], respectively; relative risk, 2.5; 95 percent confidence interval, 1.6 to 4.5). Because of these results, the part of the trial involving encainide and flecainide has been discontinued. We conclude that neither encainide nor flecainide should be used in the treatment of patients with asymptomatic or minimally symptomatic ventricular arrhythmia after myocardial infarction, even though these drugs may be effective initially in suppressing ventricular arrhythmia. Whether these results apply to other patients who might be candidates for antiarrhythmic therapy is unknown.

CAST-II Trial

Effect of the antiarrhythmic agent moricizine on survival after myocardial infarction. The Cardiac Arrhythmia Suppression Trial II Investigators.

New England Journal of Medicine (NEJM) 1992; July 23;327(4):227-33.

BACKGROUND

The Cardiac Arrhythmia Suppression Trial (CAST) tested the hypothesis that the suppression of asymptomatic or mildly symptomatic ventricular premature depolarizations in survivors of myocardial infarction would decrease the number of deaths from ventricular arrhythmias and improve overall survival. The second CAST study (CAST-II) tested this hypothesis with a comparison of moricizine and placebo.

METHODS

CAST-II was divided into two blinded, randomized phases: an early, 14-day exposure phase that evaluated the risk of starting treatment with moricizine after myocardial infarction (1325 patients), and a long-term phase that evaluated the effect of moricizine on survival after myocardial infarction in patients whose ventricular premature depolarizations were either adequately suppressed by moricizine (1155 patients) or only partially suppressed (219 patients).

RESULTS

CAST-II was stopped early because the first 14-day period of treatment with moricizine after a myocardial infarction was associated with excess mortality (17 of 665 patients died or had cardiac arrests), as compared with no treatment or placebo (3 of 660 patients died or had cardiac arrests); and estimates of conditional power indicated that it was highly unlikely (less than 8 percent chance) that a survival benefit from moricizine could be observed if the trial were completed. At the completion of the long-term phase, there were 49 deaths or cardiac arrests due to arrhythmias in patients assigned to moricizine, and 42 in patients assigned to placebo (adjusted P = 0.40).

CONCLUSIONS

As with the antiarrhythmic agents used in CAST-I (flecainide and encainide), the use of moricizine in CAST-II to suppress asymptomatic or mildly symptomatic ventricular premature depolarizations to try to reduce mortality after myocardial infarction is not only ineffective but also harmful.

SWORD TRIAL
MORTALITY IN THE SURVIVAL WITH ORAL D-SOTALOL (SWORD) TRIAL: WHY DID PATIENTS DIE?
PRATT CM ET AL.
AMERICAN JOURNAL OF CARDIOLOGY 1998: APRIL 1: 81(7):869-76.

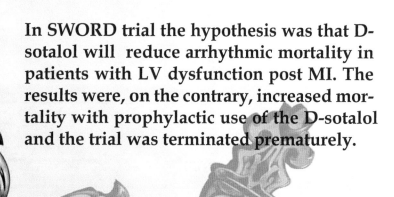

In SWORD trial the hypothesis was that D-sotalol will reduce arrhythmic mortality in patients with LV dysfunction post MI. The results were, on the contrary, increased mortality with prophylactic use of the D-sotalol and the trial was terminated prematurely.

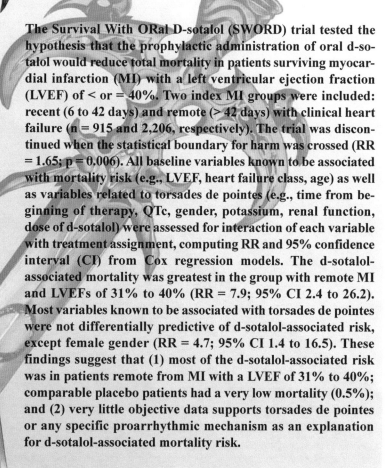

The Survival With ORal D-sotalol (SWORD) trial tested the hypothesis that the prophylactic administration of oral d-sotalol would reduce total mortality in patients surviving myocardial infarction (MI) with a left ventricular ejection fraction (LVEF) of < or = 40%. Two index MI groups were included: recent (6 to 42 days) and remote (> 42 days) with clinical heart failure (n = 915 and 2,206, respectively). The trial was discontinued when the statistical boundary for harm was crossed (RR = 1.65; p = 0.006). All baseline variables known to be associated with mortality risk (e.g., LVEF, heart failure class, age) as well as variables related to torsades de pointes (e.g., time from beginning of therapy, QTc, gender, potassium, renal function, dose of d-sotalol) were assessed for interaction of each variable with treatment assignment, computing RR and 95% confidence interval (CI) from Cox regression models. The d-sotalol-associated mortality was greatest in the group with remote MI and LVEFs of 31% to 40% (RR = 7.9; 95% CI 2.4 to 26.2). Most variables known to be associated with torsades de pointes were not differentially predictive of d-sotalol-associated risk, except female gender (RR = 4.7; 95% CI 1.4 to 16.5). These findings suggest that (1) most of the d-sotalol-associated risk was in patients remote from MI with a LVEF of 31% to 40%; comparable placebo patients had a very low mortality (0.5%); and (2) very little objective data supports torsades de pointes or any specific proarrhythmic mechanism as an explanation for d-sotalol-associated mortality risk.

CASH TRIAL
RANDOMIZED COMPARISON OF ANTIARRHYTHMIC DRUG THERAPY WITH IMPLANTABLE DEFIBRILLATORS IN PATIENTS RESUSCITATED FROM CARDIAC ARREST
CIRCULATION. 2000

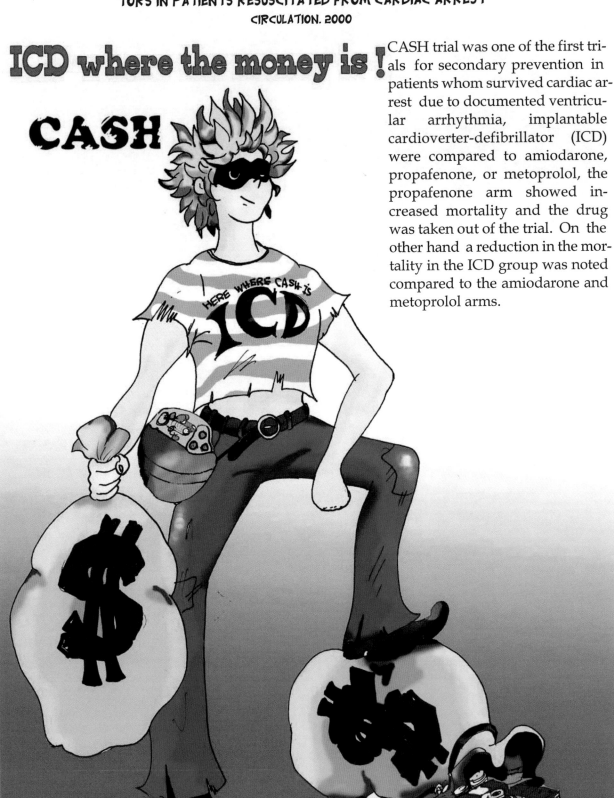

ICD where the money is !

CASH

HERE WHERE CASH IS
ICD

CASH trial was one of the first trials for secondary prevention in patients whom survived cardiac arrest due to documented ventricular arrhythmia, implantable cardioverter-defibrillator (ICD) were compared to amiodarone, propafenone, or metoprolol, the propafenone arm showed increased mortality and the drug was taken out of the trial. On the other hand a reduction in the mortality in the ICD group was noted compared to the amiodarone and metoprolol arms.

CASH Trial

Randomized comparison of antiarrhythmic drug therapy with implantable defibrillators in patients resuscitated from cardiac arrest : the Cardiac Arrest Study Hamburg (CASH). Kuck KH, et al.

Circulation. 2000; August 15;102(7):748-54.

BACKGROUND

We conducted a prospective, multicenter, randomized comparison of implantable cardioverter-defibrillator (ICD) versus antiarrhythmic drug therapy in survivors of cardiac arrest secondary to documented ventricular arrhythmias.

METHODS AND RESULTS

From 1987, eligible patients were randomized to an ICD, amiodarone, propafenone, or metoprolol (ICD versus antiarrhythmic agents randomization ratio 1:3). Assignment to propafenone was discontinued in March 1992, after an interim analysis conducted in 58 patients showed a 61% higher all-cause mortality rate than in 61 ICD patients during a follow-up of 11.3 months. The study continued to recruit 288 patients in the remaining 3 study groups; of these, 99 were assigned to ICDs, 92 to amiodarone, and 97 to metoprolol. The primary end point was all-cause mortality. The study was terminated in March 1998, when all patients had concluded a minimum 2-year follow-up. Over a mean follow-up of 57+/-34 months, the crude death rates were 36.4% (95% CI 26.9% to 46.6%) in the ICD and 44.4% (95% CI 37.2% to 51.8%) in the amiodarone/metoprolol arm. Overall survival was higher, though not significantly, in patients assigned to ICD than in those assigned to drug therapy (1-sided P=0.081, hazard ratio 0.766, [97.5% CI upper bound 1.112]). In ICD patients, the percent reductions in all-cause mortality were 41.9%, 39.3%, 28. 4%, 27.7%, 22.8%, 11.4%, 9.1%, 10.6%, and 24.7% at years 1 to 9 of follow-up.

CONCLUSIONS

During long-term follow-up of cardiac arrest survivors, therapy with an ICD is associated with a 23% (nonsignificant) reduction of all-cause mortality rates when compared with treatment with amiodarone/metoprolol. The benefit of ICD therapy is more evident during the first 5 years after the index event.

AVID AND MUSTT TRIALS

AVID trial was one of the largest secondary prevention trials. AVID looked at patients who survived cardiac VFib/VT arrest , where patients were randomized to receive ICD vs. antiarrhythmics drugs (AAD). ICD were superior in preventing arrhythmic death than AAD. While MUSTT trial was one of the first primary prevention trials, and it was designed to evaluate patients with CAD, EF 40%, and NSVT if an EP study induced sustained VT, then they were randomized to antiarrhythmic therapy (AAD) vs. no therapy, and if the AAD failed to render VT non-inducible, then ICD could be implanted. The results were decreased mortality only in patients receiving ICDs. No mortality difference were seen between the no treatment group vs. anti-arrhythmic medications group, so although the MUSTT trial was not designed to compare ICD to the AAD it demonstrated the superiority of ICD treatment vs. AAD.

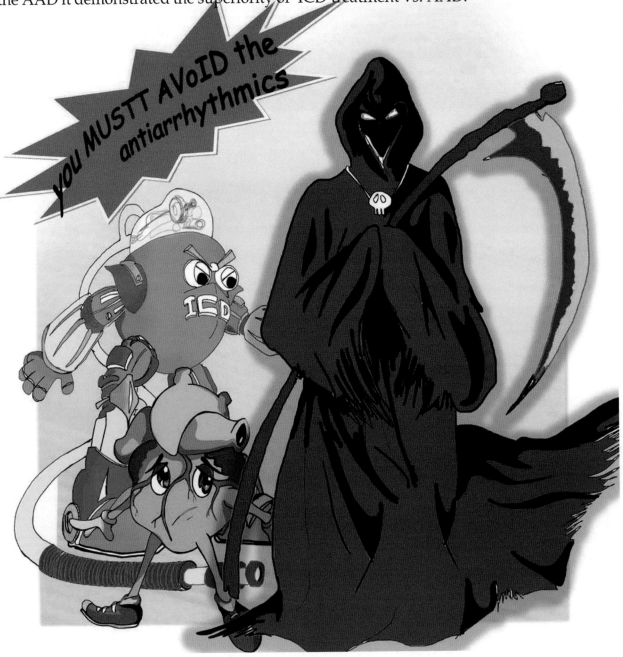

AVID Trial
Causes of death in the Antiarrhythmics Versus Implantable Defibrillators (AVID) Trial.
Journal of the American College of Cardiology (JACC) 1999; November1; 34(5):1552-9.

OBJECTIVES

This study analyzed the causes of death in the Antiarrhythmics Versus Implantable Defibrillators (AVID) Trial.

BACKGROUND

Both implantable cardioverter-defibrillators (ICDs) and antiarrhythmic drugs (AADs) are used as mainstays of treatment for life-threatening ventricular arrhythmias in patients who have survived either ventricular fibrillation or sustained ventricular tachycardia with hemodynamic compromise and serious symptoms. The AVID Trial compared the effectiveness of these two therapies. Survival was better with the ICD. Assessment of the cause of death should help to determine the mechanism of improvement in survival with the ICD.

METHODS

Of 1,016 patients enrolled in the AVID Trial, 202 patients died. The mode of death was determined by the unblinded Principal Investigator and independently by an Events Committee, which reviewed materials meticulously blinded with respect to treatment. Deaths were classified as cardiac or noncardiac. Cardiac deaths were further classified as arrhythmic or nonarrhythmic, and causes of noncardiac death were identified.

RESULTS

Deaths were more frequent in patients treated with an AAD (n = 122), compared with patients treated with the ICD (n = 80), unadjusted p < 0.001, p = 0.012 adjusted for sequential monitoring. In AVID, 157 deaths were cardiac, and 79 were arrhythmic. The major effect of the ICD was to prevent arrhythmic death (AAD = 55, ICD = 24, nominal unadjusted p < 0.001). Nonarrhythmic cardiac deaths were equal (AAD = 39, ICD = 39). Patients treated with an AAD had a slightly greater incidence of noncardiac deaths (28 vs. 17, p = 0.053), primarily due to pulmonary and renal causes.

CONCLUSIONS

The ICD is more effective than an AAD in reducing arrhythmic cardiac death, while nonarrhythmic cardiac death is unchanged. Of note, apparent arrhythmic death still seems to constitute 38% of all cardiac deaths despite treatment with an ICD. However, the ICD remains superior to an AAD in prolonging survival after life-threatening arrhythmias

MUSTT Trial
A RANDOMIZED STUDY OF THE PREVENTION OF SUDDEN DEATH IN PATIENTS WITH CORONARY ARTERY DISEASE. BUXTON, A et al.
New England Journal of Medicine (NEJM) 1999, December 16; 341:1882-1890.

BACKGROUND

Empirical antiarrhythmic therapy has not reduced mortality among patients with coronary artery disease and asymptomatic ventricular arrhythmias. Previous studies have suggested that antiarrhythmic therapy guided by electrophysiologic testing might reduce the risk of sudden death.

METHODS

We conducted a randomized, controlled trial to test the hypothesis that electrophysiologically guided antiarrhythmic therapy would reduce the risk of sudden death among patients with coronary artery disease, a left ventricular ejection fraction of 40 percent or less, and asymptomatic, unsustained ventricular tachycardia. Patients in whom sustained ventricular tachyarrhythmias were induced by programmed stimulation were randomly assigned to receive either antiarrhythmic therapy, including drugs and implantable defibrillators, as indicated by the results of electrophysiologic testing, or no antiarrhythmic therapy. Angiotensin-converting–enzyme inhibitors and beta-adrenergic–blocking agents were administered if the patients could tolerate them.

RESULTS

A total of 704 patients with inducible, sustained ventricular tachyarrhythmias were randomly assigned to treatment groups. Five-year Kaplan–Meier estimates of the incidence of the primary end point of cardiac arrest or death from arrhythmia were 25 percent among those receiving electrophysiologically guided therapy and 32 percent among the patients assigned to no antiarrhythmic therapy (relative risk, 0.73; 95 percent confidence interval, 0.53 to 0.99), representing a reduction in risk of 27 percent. The five-year estimates of overall mortality were 42 percent and 48 percent, respectively (relative risk, 0.80; 95 percent confidence interval, 0.64 to 1.01). The risk of cardiac arrest or death from arrhythmia among the patients who received treatment with defibrillators was significantly lower than that among the patients discharged without receiving defibrillator treatment (relative risk, 0.24; 95 percent confidence interval, 0.13 to 0.45; P<0.001). Neither the rate of cardiac arrest or death from arrhythmia nor the overall mortality rate was lower among the patients assigned to electrophysiologically guided therapy and treated with antiarrhythmic drugs than among the patients assigned to no antiarrhythmic therapy.

CONCLUSIONS

Electrophysiologically guided antiarrhythmic therapy with implantable defibrillators, but not with antiarrhythmic drugs, reduces the risk of sudden death in high-risk patients with coronary disease.

MADIT AND MADIT-II TRIALS
MULTICENTER AUTOMATIC DEFIBRILLATOR IMPLANTATION TRIAL

The MADIT trials were one of the first trials in primary prevention of sudden cardiac death. The MADIT-I showed that the implantable cardioverter defibrillator (ICD) saves lives in high-risk patients with coronary heart disease, and positive EPS for inducible ventricular arrhythmia. MADIT-II study showed that prophylactic ICD therapy was associated with significantly improved survival in patients with ischemic cardiomyopathy and advanced left ventricular dysfunction, without requiring screening for ventricular arrhythmias or inducibility by electrophysiologic testing.

With the aid of the ICDs .. the hearts were able to MADE IT

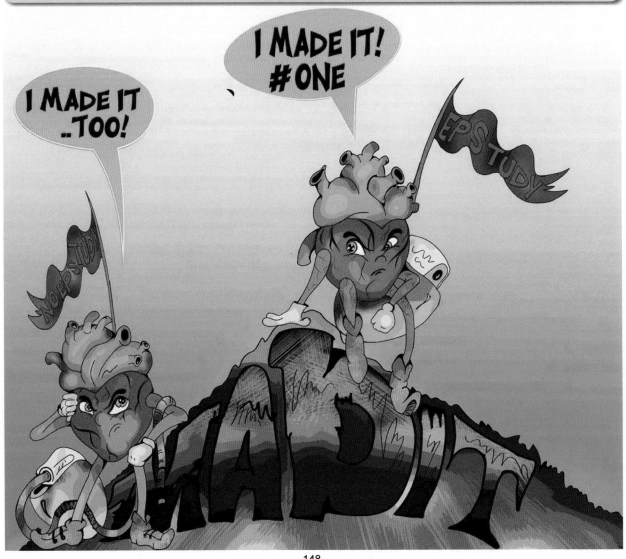

MADIT

Improved survival with an implanted defibrillator in patients with coronary disease at high risk for ventricular arrhythmia. Multicenter Automatic Defibrillator Implantation Trial Investigators. Moss AJ,

New England Journal of Medicine (NEJM) 1996; December 26; 335(26):1933-40.

BACKGROUND

Unsustained ventricular tachycardia in patients with previous myocardial infarction and left ventricular dysfunction is associated with a two-year mortality rate of about 30 percent. We studied whether prophylactic therapy with an implanted cardioverter-defibrillator, as compared with conventional medical therapy, would improve survival in this high-risk group of patients.

METHODS

Over the course of five years, 196 patients in New York Heart Association functional class I, II, or III with prior myocardial infarction; a left ventricular ejection fraction < or = 0.35; a documented episode of asymptomatic unsustained ventricular tachycardia; and inducible, nonsuppressible ventricular tachyarrhythmia on electrophysiologic study were randomly assigned to receive an implanted defibrillator (n = 95) or conventional medical therapy (n=101). We used a two-sided sequential design with death from any cause as the end point.

RESULTS

The base-line characteristics of the two treatment groups were similar. During an average follow-up of 27 months, there were 15 deaths in the defibrillator group (11 from cardiac causes) and 39 deaths in the conventional-therapy group (27 from cardiac causes) (hazard ratio for overall mortality, 0.46; 95 percent confidence interval, 0.26 to 0.82; P=0.009). There was no evidence that amiodarone, beta-blockers, or any other antiarrhythmic therapy had a significant influence on the observed hazard ratio.

CONCLUSIONS

In patients with a prior myocardial infarction who are at high risk for ventricular tachyarrhythmia, prophylactic therapy with an implanted defibrillator leads to improved survival as compared with conventional medical therapy.

MADIT-II

Prophylactic implantation of a defibrillator in patients with myocardial infarction and reduced ejection fraction.

Moss AJ, et al. Multicenter Automatic Defibrillator ImplantationTrial II Investigators.

New England Journal of Medicine (NEJM) 2002 March 21;346(12):877-83.

BACKGROUND

Patients with reduced left ventricular function after myocardial infarction are at risk for life-threatening ventricular arrhythmias. This randomized trial was designed to evaluate the effect of an implantable defibrillator on survival in such patients.

METHODS

Over the course of four years, we enrolled 1232 patients with a prior myocardial infarction and a left ventricular ejection fraction of 0.30 or less. Patients were randomly assigned in a 3:2 ratio to receive an implantable defibrillator (742 patients) or conventional medical therapy (490 patients). Invasive electrophysiological testing for risk stratification was not required. Death from any cause was the end point.

RESULTS

The clinical characteristics at base line and the prevalence of medication use at the time of the last follow-up visit were similar in the two treatment groups. During an average follow-up of 20 months, the mortality rates were 19.8 percent in the conventional-therapy group and 14.2 percent in the defibrillator group. The hazard ratio for the risk of death from any cause in the defibrillator group as compared with the conventional-therapy group was 0.69 (95 percent confidence interval, 0.51 to 0.93; P=0.016). The effect of defibrillator therapy on survival was similar in subgroup analyses stratified according to age, sex, ejection fraction, New York Heart Association class, and the QRS interval.

CONCLUSIONS

In patients with a prior myocardial infarction and advanced left ventricular dysfunction, prophylactic implantation of a defibrillatorimproves survival and should be considered as a recommended therapy.

SUDDEN CARDIAC DEATH IN HEART FAILURE TRIAL (SCD-HEFT) AMIODARONE OR AN IMPLANTABLE CARDIOVERTER-DEFIBRILLATOR FOR CONGESTIVE HEART FAILURE.

SCD-HeFT was one of the first trials that confirmed the effectiveness of the ICD in patients with non-ischemic cardiomyopathy, in addition to patients with ischemic cardiomyopathy, to decrease overall mortality . While amiodarone was comparable to placebo in terms of survival benefits. The previous trials (MADIT trials and MUSTT) included only patients with history of ischemic cardiomyopathy.

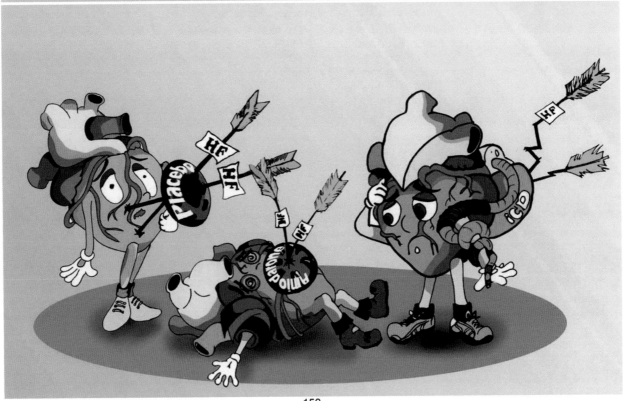

The Hearts are SUDDENLY dying with the heart failure arrows .. nothing seems to protect except for the ICD shields

CAT TRIAL
PRIMARY PREVENTION OF SUDDEN CARDIAC DEATH IN IDIOPATHIC DILATED CARDIOMYOPATHY: THE CARDIOMYOPATHY TRIAL (CAT).

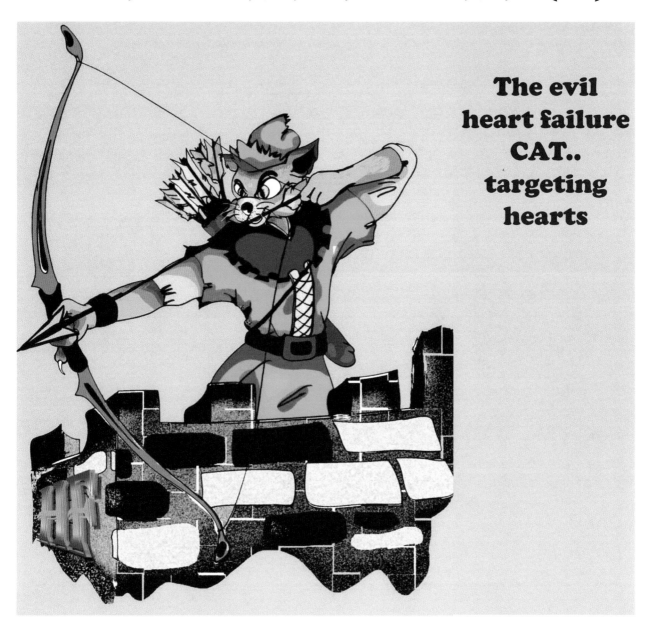

The evil heart failure CAT.. targeting hearts

CAT trial was conducted in patients with non-ischemic cardiomyopathy, and it was done prior to SCD-HeFT trial. This trial failed to show mortality benefit using ICD in this population. CAT trial, however, was a small trial and was terminated early due to low incidence rate of end-point (all –cause mortality) in the control group.

SCD-HeFT Trial

Amiodarone or an implantable cardioverter-defibrillator for congestive heart failure.
Bardy GH et al. Sudden Cardiac Death in Heart Failure Trial (SCD-HeFT) Investigators.

New England Journal of Medicine (NEJM) 2005 January 20; 352(3):225-37.

BACKGROUND

Sudden death from cardiac causes remains a leading cause of death among patients with congestive heart failure (CHF). Treatment with amiodarone or an implantable cardioverter-defibrillator (ICD) has been proposed to improve the prognosis in such patients.

METHODS

We randomly assigned 2521 patients with New York Heart Association (NYHA) class II or III CHF and a left ventricular ejection fraction (LVEF) of 35 percent or less to conventional therapy for CHF plus placebo (847 patients), conventional therapy plus amiodarone (845 patients), or conventional therapy plus a conservatively programmed, shock-only, single-lead ICD (829 patients). Placebo and amiodarone were administered in a double-blind fashion. The primary end point was death from any cause.

RESULTS

The median LVEF in patients was 25 percent; 70 percent were in NYHA class II, and 30 percent were in class III CHF. The cause of CHF was ischemic in 52 percent and nonischemic in 48 percent. The median follow-up was 45.5 months. There were 244 deaths (29 percent) in the placebo group, 240 (28 percent) in the amiodarone group, and 182 (22 percent) in the ICD group. As compared with placebo, amiodarone was associated with a similar risk of death (hazard ratio, 1.06; 97.5 percent confidence interval, 0.86 to 1.30; P=0.53) and ICD therapy was associated with a decreased risk of death of 23 percent (0.77; 97.5 percent confidence interval, 0.62 to 0.96; P=0.007) and an absolute decrease in mortality of 7.2 percentage points after five years in the overall population. Results did not vary according to either ischemic or nonischemic causes of CHF, but they did vary according to the NYHA class.

CONCLUSIONS

In patients with NYHA class II or III CHF and LVEF of 35 percent or less, amiodarone has no favorable effect on survival, whereas single-lead, shock-only ICD therapy reduces overall mortality by 23 percent.

CAT Trial

Primary prevention of sudden cardiac death in idiopathic dilated cardiomyopathy: the Cardiomyopathy Trial (CAT).Bänsch D, et al.

Circulation. 2002 March 26;105(12):1453-8.

BACKGROUND

Patients with idiopathic dilated cardiomyopathy (DCM) and impaired left ventricular ejection fraction have an increased risk of dying suddenly.

METHODS AND RESULTS

Patients with recent onset of DCM (< or =9 months) and an ejection fraction < or =30% were randomly assigned to the implantation of an implantable cardioverter-defibrillator (ICD) or control. The primary end point of the trial was all-cause mortality at 1 year of follow-up. The trial was terminated after the inclusion of 104 patients because the all-cause mortality rate at 1 year did not reach the expected 30% in the control group. In August 2000, the vital status of all patients was updated by contacting patients, relatives, or local registration offices. One hundred four patients were enrolled in the trial: Fifty were assigned to ICD therapy and 54 to the control group. Mean follow-up was 22.8+/-4.3 months, on the basis of investigators' follow-up. After 1 year, 6 patients were dead (4 in the ICD group and 2 in the control group). No sudden death occurred during the first and second years of follow-up. In August 2000, after a mean follow-up of 5.5+/-2.2 years, 30 deaths had occurred (13 in the ICD group and 17 in the control group). Cumulative survival was not significantly different between the two groups (93% and 80% in the control group versus 92% and 86% in the ICD group after 2 and 4 years, respectively).

CONCLUSIONS

This trial did not provide evidence in favor of prophylactic ICD implantation in patients with DCM of recent onset and impaired left ventricular ejection fraction.

DINAMIT AND IRIS TRIALS
PROPHYLACTIC USE OF AN IMPLANTABLE CARDIOVERTER–DEFIBRILLATOR AFTER ACUTE MYOCARDIAL INFARCTION.

The DINAMIT and the IRIS trials looked at patients with recent myocardial infract (less than 40, and 30 days post MI, respectively). No significant decrease in all-cause mortality in patients receiving ICDs in both trials, although IRIS showed decreased incidence of sudden cardiac death in the ICD arm.

ICD FAILED ..WALK OF SHAME

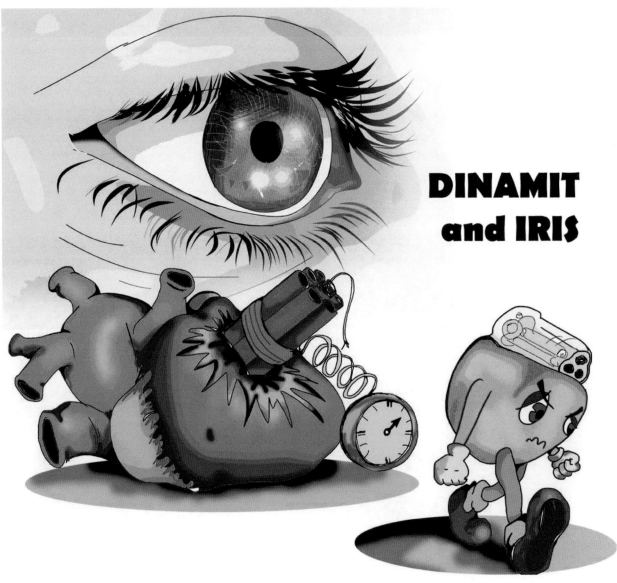

DINAMIT and IRIS

DINAMIT

Prophylactic Use of an Implantable Cardioverter-Defibrillator after Acute Myocardial Infarction. Stefan H. et al. for the DINAMIT Investigators

New England Journal of Medicine (NEJM) 2004, December 9; 351:2481-2488.

BACKGROUND

Implantable cardioverter-defibrillator (ICD) therapy has been shown to improve survival in patients with various heart conditions who are at high risk for ventricular arrhythmias. Whether benefit occurs in patients early after myocardial infarction is unknown.

METHODS

We conducted the Defibrillator in Acute Myocardial Infarction Trial, a randomized, open-label comparison of ICD therapy (in 332 patients) and no ICD therapy (in 342 patients) 6 to 40 days after a myocardial infarction. We enrolled patients who had reduced left ventricular function (left ventricular ejection fraction, 0.35 or less) and impaired cardiac autonomic function (manifested as depressed heart-rate variability or an elevated average 24-hour heart rate on Holter monitoring). The primary outcome was mortality from any cause. Death from arrhythmia was a predefined secondary outcome.

RESULTS

During a mean ($\pm$SD) follow-up period of 30$\pm$13 months, there was no difference in overall mortality between the two treatment groups: of the 120 patients who died, 62 were in the ICD group and 58 in the control group (hazard ratio for death in the ICD group, 1.08; 95 percent confidence interval, 0.76 to 1.55; P=0.66). There were 12 deaths due to arrhythmia in the ICD group, as compared with 29 in the control group (hazard ratio in the ICD group, 0.42; 95 percent confidence interval, 0.22 to 0.83; P=0.009). In contrast, there were 50 deaths from nonarrhythmic causes in the ICD group and 29 in the control group (hazard ratio in the ICD group, 1.75; 95 percent confidence interval, 1.11 to 2.76; P=0.02).

CONCLUSIONS

Prophylactic ICD therapy does not reduce overall mortality in high-risk patients who have recently had a myocardial infarction. Although ICD therapy was associated with a reduction in the rate of death due to arrhythmia, that was offset by an increase in the rate of death from nonarrhythmic causes.

IRIS

Defibrillator implantation early after myocardial infarction. Steinbeck G, et al. IRIS Investigators.

New England Journal of Medicine (NEJM) 2009 October 8;361(15):1427-36.

BACKGROUND

The rate of death, including sudden cardiac death, is highest early after a myocardial infarction. Yet current guidelines do not recommend the use of an implantable cardioverter-defibrillator (ICD) within 40 days after a myocardial infarction for the prevention of sudden cardiac death. We tested the hypothesis that patients at increased risk who are treated early with an ICD will live longer than those who receive optimal medical therapy alone.

METHODS

This randomized, prospective, open-label, investigator-initiated, multicenter trial registered 62,944 unselected patients with myocardial infarction. Of this total, 898 patients were enrolled 5 to 31 days after the event if they met certain clinical criteria: a reduced left ventricular ejection fraction (< or = 40%) and a heart rate of 90 or more beats per minute on the first available electrocardiogram (ECG) (criterion 1: 602 patients), nonsustained ventricular tachycardia (> or = 150 beats per minute) during Holter monitoring (criterion 2: 208 patients), or both criteria (88 patients). Of the 898 patients, 445 were randomly assigned to treatment with an ICD and 453 to medical therapy alone.

RESULTS

During a mean follow-up of 37 months, 233 patients died: 116 patients in the ICD group and 117 patients in the control group. Overall mortality was not reduced in the ICD group (hazard ratio, 1.04; 95% confidence interval [CI], 0.81 to 1.35; P=0.78). There were fewer sudden cardiac deaths in the ICD group than in the control group (27 vs. 60; hazard ratio, 0.55; 95% CI, 0.31 to 1.00; P=0.049), but the number of nonsudden cardiac deaths was higher (68 vs. 39; hazard ratio, 1.92; 95% CI, 1.29 to 2.84; P=0.001). Hazard ratios were similar among the three groups of patients categorized according to the enrollment criteria they met (criterion 1, criterion 2, or both).

CONCLUSIONS

Prophylactic ICD therapy did not reduce overall mortality among patients with acute myocardial infarction and clinical features that placed them at increased risk.

MUSTIC TRIAL
EFFECTS OF MULTISITE BIVENTRICULAR PACING IN PATIENTS WITH HEART FAILURE AND INTRAVENTRICULAR CONDUCTION DELAY.
NEW ENGLAND JOURNAL OF MEDICINE (NEJM) 2001.

MUSTIC study was one of the early studies (along with MIRACLE trial) to show the potential benefit of Cardiac Resynchronization with Biventricular pacing in patients with CHF with intraventricular conduction delay CRT was associated with improvement in both exercise tolerance and quality of life. Later on CARE-HF showed also that CRT was associated with lower mortality in this group.

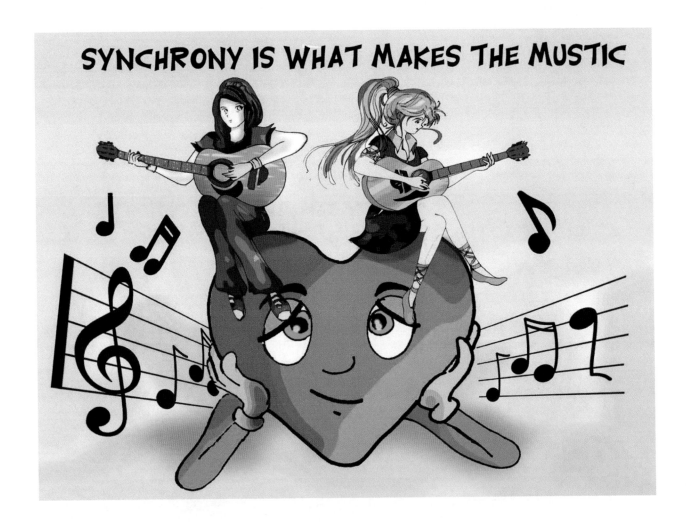

MUSTIC TRIAL
Effects of multisite biventricular pacing in patients with heart failure and intraventricular conduction delay.
Cazeau S et al.
New England Journal of Medicine (NEJM) 2001; March 22;344(12):873-80.

BACKGROUND:

One third of patients with chronic heart failure have electrocardiographic evidence of a major intraventricular conduction delay, which may worsen left ventricular systolic dysfunction through asynchronous ventricular contraction. Uncontrolled studies suggest that multisite biventricular pacing improves hemodynamics and well-being by reducing ventricular asynchrony. We assessed the clinical efficacy and safety of this new therapy.

METHODS:

Sixty-seven patients with severe heart failure (New York Heart Association class III) due to chronic left ventricular systolic dysfunction, with normal sinus rhythm and a duration of the QRS interval of more than 150 msec, received transvenous atriobiventricular pacemakers (with leads in one atrium and each ventricle). This single-blind, randomized, controlled crossover study compared the responses of the patients during two periods: a three-month period of inactive pacing (ventricular inhibited pacing at a basic rate of 40 bpm) and a three-month period of active (atriobiventricular) pacing. The primary end point was the distance walked in six minutes; the secondary end points were the quality of life as measured by questionnaire, peak oxygen consumption, hospitalizations related to heart failure, the patients' treatment preference (active vs. inactive pacing), and the mortality rate.

RESULTS:

Nine patients were withdrawn from the study before randomization, and 10 failed to complete both study periods. Thus, 48 patients completed both phases of the study. The mean distance walked in six minutes was 22 percent greater with active pacing (399+/-100 m vs. 326+/-134 m, P<0.001), the quality-of-life score improved by 32 percent (P<0.001), peak oxygen uptake increased by 8 percent (P<0.03), hospitalizations were decreased by two thirds (P<0.05), and active pacing was preferred by 85 percent of the patients (P<0.001).

CONCLUSIONS:

Although it is technically complex, atriobiventricular pacing significantly improves exercise tolerance and quality of life in patients with chronic heart failure and intraventricular conduction delay.

MIRACLE AND CARE-HF TRIALS

MIRACLE was one of the first trials to demonstrate clinical benefit from BiV pacing vs. no pacing . Patient population in this trial were of moderate-to-severe heart failure, and they showed improved clinical symptoms and less heart failure hospitalization. CARE-HF showed that cardiac resynchronization therapy CRT did not only improve the symptoms and quality of life in patients with heart failure, as it was found with MUSTIC and MIRACLE trials, but it was also associated with a survival benefits as well..

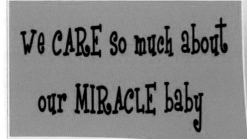

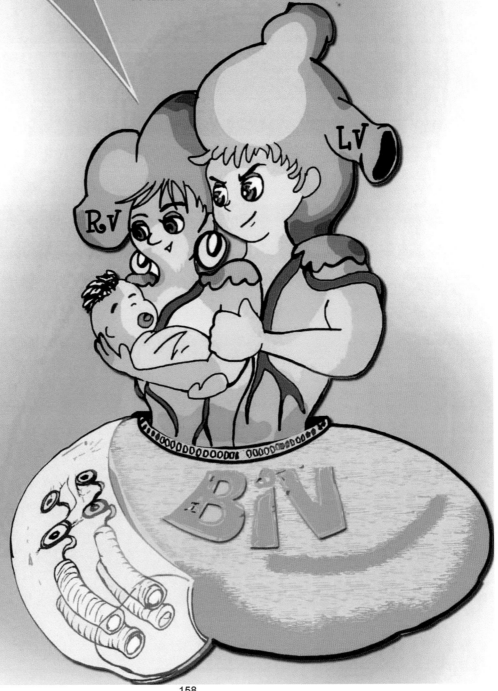

158

MIRACLE TRIAL
Cardiac Resynchronization in Chronic Heart Failure
William T. Abraham, M.D et al.
New England Journal of Medicine (NEJM) 2002; June 13, 346:1845-1853.

BACKGROUND

Previous studies have suggested that cardiac resynchronization achieved through atrial-synchronized biventricular pacing produces clinical benefits in patients with heart failure who have an intraventricular conduction delay. We conducted a double-blind trial to evaluate this therapeutic approach.

METHODS

Four hundred fifty-three patients with moderate-to-severe symptoms of heart failure associated with an ejection fraction of 35 percent or less and a QRS interval of 130 msec or more were randomly assigned to a cardiac-resynchronization group (228 patients) or to a control group (225 patients) for six months, while conventional therapy for heart failure was maintained. The primary end points were the New York Heart Association functional class, quality of life, and the distance walked in six minutes.

RESULTS

As compared with the control group, patients assigned to cardiac resynchronization experienced an improvement in the distance walked in six minutes (+39 vs. +10 m, P=0.005), functional class (P<0.001), quality of life (–18.0 vs. –9.0 points, P= 0.001), time on the treadmill during exercise testing (+81 vs. +19 sec, P=0.001), and ejection fraction (+4.6 percent vs. –0.2 percent, P<0.001). In addition, fewer patients in the group assigned to cardiac resynchronization than control patients required hospitalization (8 percent vs. 15 percent) or intravenous medications (7 percent vs. 15 percent) for the treatment of heart failure (P<0.05 for both comparisons). Implantation of the device was unsuccessful in 8 percent of patients and was complicated by refractory hypotension, bradycardia, or asystole in four patients (two of whom died) and by perforation of the coronary sinus requiring pericardiocentesis in two others.

CONCLUSIONS

Cardiac resynchronization results in significant clinical improvement in patients who have moderate-to-severe heart failure and an intraventricular conduction delay.

CARE-HF TRIAL
The Effect of Cardiac Resynchronization on Morbidity and Mortality in Heart Failure.
John G.F et al.
New England Journal of Medicine (NEJM) 2005; April 14, 352:1539-1549.

BACKGROUND

Cardiac resynchronization reduces symptoms and improves left ventricular function in many patients with heart failure due to left ventricular systolic dysfunction and cardiac dyssynchrony. We evaluated its effects on morbidity and mortality.

METHODS

Patients with New York Heart Association class III or IV heart failure due to left ventricular systolic dysfunction and cardiac dyssynchrony who were receiving standard pharmacologic therapy were randomly assigned to receive medical therapy alone or with cardiac resynchronization. The primary end point was the time to death from any cause or an unplanned hospitalization for a major cardiovascular event. The principal secondary end point was death from any cause.

RESULTS

A total of 813 patients were enrolled and followed for a mean of 29.4 months. The primary end point was reached by 159 patients in the cardiac-resynchronization group, as compared with 224 patients in the medical-therapy group (39 percent vs. 55 percent; hazard ratio, 0.63; 95 percent confidence interval, 0.51 to 0.77; P<0.001). There were 82 deaths in the cardiac-resynchronization group, as compared with 120 in the medical-therapy group (20 percent vs. 30 percent; hazard ratio 0.64; 95 percent confidence interval, 0.48 to 0.85; P<0.002). As compared with medical therapy, cardiac resynchronization reduced the interventricular mechanical delay, the end-systolic volume index, and the area of the mitral regurgitant jet; increased the left ventricular ejection fraction; and improved symptoms and the quality of life (P<0.01 for all comparisons).

CONCLUSIONS

In patients with heart failure and cardiac dyssynchrony, cardiac resynchronization improves symptoms and the quality of life and reduces complications and the risk of death. These benefits are in addition to those afforded by standard pharmacologic therapy. The implantation of a cardiac-resynchronization device should routinely be considered in such patients.

COMPANION TRIAL

CARDIAC-RESYNCHRONIZATION THERAPY WITH OR WITHOUT AN IMPLANTABLE DEFIBRILLATOR IN ADVANCED CHRONIC HEART FAILURE
NEW ENGLAND JOURNAL OF MEDICINE (NEJM) 2004.

The COMPANION trial is one of the largest heart failure device trials, it showed that cardiac re-synchronization therapy (CRT), used in combination with optimal pharmacologic therapy (OPT) , can significantly improve both the quality and duration of life for a large group of heart failure patients. The cardiac resynchronization therapy with defibrillator capacity (CRT-D) in combination with optimal pharmacologic therapy significantly reduced the risk of all cause mortality compared to OPT alone . The mortality reduction in the resynchronization-alone without defibrillator capacity was approximately half the reduction in the resynchronization/ICD group.

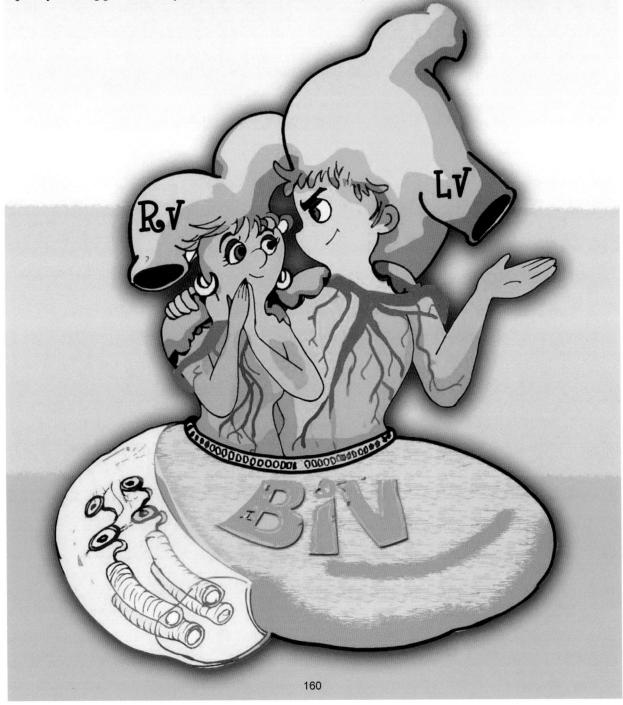

Companion trial
Cardiac-Resynchronization Therapy with or without an Implantable Defibrillator in Advanced Chronic Heart Failure
Michael R. et al.

New England Journal of Medicine (NEJM) 2004; May 20; 350:2140-2150 .

BACKGROUND

We tested the hypothesis that prophylactic cardiac-resynchronization therapy in the form of biventricular stimulation with a pacemaker with or without a defibrillator would reduce the risk of death and hospitalization among patients with advanced chronic heart failure and intraventricular conduction delays.

METHODS

A total of 1520 patients who had advanced heart failure (New York Heart Association class III or IV) due to ischemic or nonischemic cardiomyopathies and a QRS interval of at least 120 msec were randomly assigned in a 1:2:2 ratio to receive optimal pharmacologic therapy (diuretics, angiotensin-converting–enzyme inhibitors, beta-blockers, and spironolactone) alone or in combination with cardiac-resynchronization therapy with either a pacemaker or a pacemaker–defibrillator. The primary composite end point was the time to death from or hospitalization for any cause.

RESULTS

As compared with optimal pharmacologic therapy alone, cardiac-resynchronization therapy with a pacemaker decreased the risk of the primary end point (hazard ratio, 0.81; P=0.014), as did cardiac-resynchronization therapy with a pacemaker–defibrillator (hazard ratio, 0.80; P=0.01). The risk of the combined end point of death from or hospitalization for heart failure was reduced by 34 percent in the pacemaker group (P<0.002) and by 40 percent in the pacemaker–defibrillator group (P<0.001 for the comparison with the pharmacologic-therapy group). A pacemaker reduced the risk of the secondary end point of death from any cause by 24 percent (P=0.059), and a pacemaker–defibrillator reduced the risk by 36 percent (P=0.003).

CONCLUSIONS

In patients with advanced heart failure and a prolonged QRS interval, cardiac-resynchronization therapy decreases the combined risk of death from any cause or first hospitalization and, when combined with an implantable defibrillator, significantly reduces mortality.

MADIT-CRT
CARDIAC-RESYNCHRONIZATION THERAPY FOR THE PREVENTION OF HEART-FAILURE EVENTS

THE NEW ENGLAND JOURNAL OF MEDICINE (NEJM) 2009.

CRT therapy established benefits in patients with New York Heart Association(NYHA) class III-IV symptoms. The MADIT-CRT proved that the CRT therapy is also beneficial in patients with New York Heart Association class I or II symptoms, so asymptomatic heart failure patients with wide QRS (>150 ms) showed less heart failure events when treated with CRT vs. medical therapy. However, mortality was comparable between the two groups.

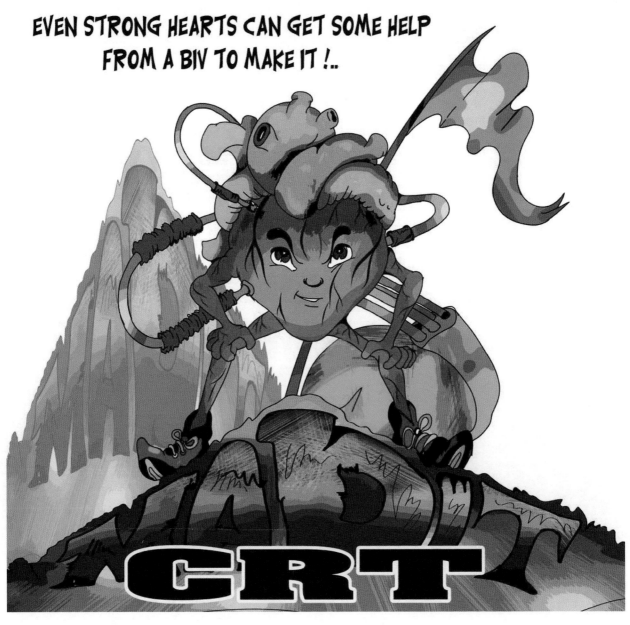

MADIT-CRT

Cardiac-Resynchronization Therapy for the Prevention of Heart-Failure Events
Arthur J. Moss, et al

New England Journal of Medicine (NEJM) 2009; October 1, 361:1329-1338

BACKGROUND:

This trial was designed to determine whether cardiac-resynchronization therapy (CRT) with biventricular pacing would reduce the risk of death or heart-failure events in patients with mild cardiac symptoms, a reduced ejection fraction, and a wide QRS complex.

METHODS:

During a 4.5-year period, we enrolled and followed 1820 patients with ischemic or nonischemic cardiomyopathy, an ejection fraction of 30% or less, a QRS duration of 130 msec or more, and New York Heart Association class I or II symptoms. Patients were randomly assigned in a 3:2 ratio to receive CRT plus an implantable cardioverter-defibrillator (ICD) (1089 patients) or an ICD alone (731 patients). The primary end point was death from any cause or a nonfatal heart-failure event (whichever came first). Heart-failure events were diagnosed by physicians who were aware of the treatment assignments, but they were adjudicated by a committee that was unaware of assignments.

RESULTS:

During an average follow-up of 2.4 years, the primary end point occurred in 187 of 1089 patients in the CRT-ICD group (17.2%) and 185 of 731 patients in the ICD-only group (25.3%) (hazard ratio in the CRT-ICD group, 0.66; 95% confidence interval [CI], 0.52 to 0.84; P=0.001). The benefit did not differ significantly between patients with ischemic cardiomyopathy and those with nonischemic cardiomyopathy. The superiority of CRT was driven by a 41% reduction in the risk of heart-failure events, a finding that was evident primarily in a prespecified subgroup of patients with a QRS duration of 150 msec or more. CRT was associated with a significant reduction in left ventricular volumes and improvement in the ejection fraction. There was no significant difference between the two groups in the overall risk of death, with a 3% annual mortality rate in each treatment group. Serious adverse events were infrequent in the two groups.

CONCLUSIONS:

CRT combined with ICD decreased the risk of heart-failure events in relatively asymptomatic patients with a low ejection fraction and wide QRS complex.

CTOPP TRIAL
EFFECTS OF PHYSIOLOGIC PACING VERSUS VENTRICULAR PACING ON THE RISK OF STROKE AND DEATH DUE TO CARDIOVASCULAR CAUSES.
CANADIAN TRIAL OF PHYSIOLOGIC PACING INVESTIGATORS.
NEJM 2000

CTOPP trail was one of the first trials to show the benefit of atrioventricular (AV) Pacing (Dual Chambers Pacers) over solely ventricular pacing (VVI). AV sequential pacing was associated with reduction in rate of atrial fibrillation, stroke and death.

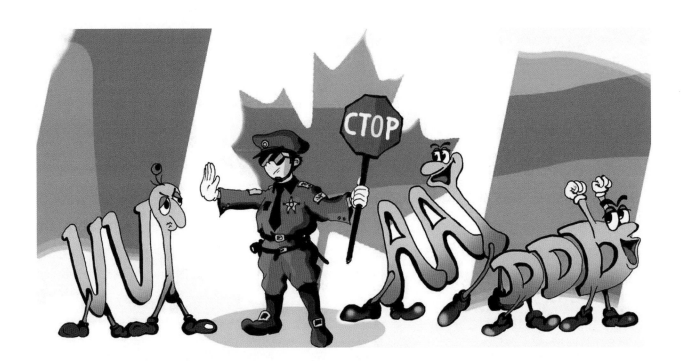

CTOPP Trial
Effects of physiologic pacing versus ventricular pacing on the risk of stroke and death due to cardiovascular causes.
Canadian Trial of Physiologic Pacing Investigators. Connolly SJ, et al

The New England Journal of Medicine (NEJM) 2000; May 11; 342(19):1385-91.

BACKGROUND:

Evidence suggests that physiologic pacing (dual-chamber or atrial) may be superior to single-chamber (ventricular) pacing because it is associated with lower risks of atrial fibrillation, stroke, and death. These benefits have not been evaluated in a large, randomized, controlled trial.

METHODS:

At 32 Canadian centers, patients without chronic atrial fibrillation who were scheduled for a first implantation of a pacemaker to treat symptomatic bradycardia were eligible for enrollment. We randomly assigned patients to receive either a ventricular pacemaker or a physiologic pacemaker and followed them for an average of three years. The primary outcome was stroke or death due to cardiovascular causes. Secondary outcomes were death from any cause, atrial fibrillation, and hospitalization for heart failure.

RESULTS:

A total of 1474 patients were randomly assigned to receive a ventricular pacemaker and 1094 to receive a physiologic pacemaker. The annual rate of stroke or death due to cardiovascular causes was 5.5 percent with ventricular pacing, as compared with 4.9 percent with physiologic pacing (reduction in relative risk, 9.4 percent; 95 percent confidence interval, -10.5 to 25.7 percent [the negative value indicates an increase in risk]; $P=0.33$). The annual rate of atrial fibrillation was significantly lower among the patients in the physiologic-pacing group (5.3 percent) than among those in the ventricular-pacing group (6.6 percent), for a reduction in relative risk of 18.0 percent (95 percent confidence interval, 0.3 to 32.6 percent; $P=0.05$). The effect on the rate of atrial fibrillation was not apparent until two years after implantation. The observed annual rates of death from all causes and of hospitalization for heart failure were lower among the patients with a physiologic pacemaker than among those with a ventricular pacemaker, but not significantly so (annual rates of death, 6.6 percent with ventricular pacing and 6.3 percent with physiologic pacing; annual rates of hospitalization for heart failure, 3.5 percent and 3.1 percent, respectively). There were significantly more perioperative complications with physiologic pacing than with ventricular pacing (9.0 percent vs. 3.8 percent, $P<0.001$).

CONCLUSIONS:

Physiologic pacing provides little benefit over ventricular pacing for the prevention of stroke or death due to cardiovascular causes.

MOST TRIAL

VENTRICULAR PACING OR DUAL-CHAMBER PACING FOR SINUS-NODE DYSFUNCTION
NEW ENGLAND JOURNAL OF MEDICINE (NEJM) 2002.

As CTOPP showed the potential benefit of Dual-Chamber Pacing over ventricular pacing in patients with bradycardia, MOST showed that was the case in patients with sinus-node dysfunction. The difference was that in MOST DDD was only associated with reduction in atrial fibrillation and improvement in symptoms and quality of life without a reduction in stroke.

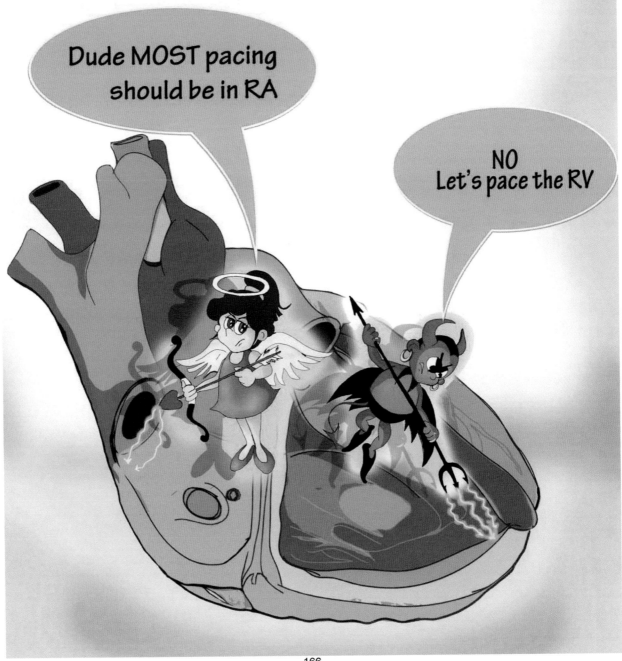

MOST TRIAL
Ventricular Pacing or Dual-Chamber Pacing for Sinus-Node Dysfunction
Gervasio A. Lamas, et al.
New England Journal of Medicine (NEJM) 2002; June 13; 346:1854-1862

BACKGROUND

Dual-chamber (atrioventricular) and single-chamber (ventricular) pacing are alternative treatment approaches for sinus-node dysfunction that causes clinically significant bradycardia. However, it is unknown which type of pacing results in the better outcome.

METHODS

We randomly assigned a total of 2010 patients with sinus-node dysfunction to dual-chamber pacing (1014 patients) or ventricular pacing (996 patients) and followed them for a median of 33.1 months. The primary end point was death from any cause or nonfatal stroke. Secondary end points included the composite of death, stroke, or hospitalization for heart failure; atrial fibrillation; heart-failure score; the pacemaker syndrome; and the quality of life.

RESULTS

The incidence of the primary end point did not differ significantly between the dual-chamber group (21.5 percent) and the ventricular-paced group (23.0 percent, P=0.48). In patients assigned to dual-chamber pacing, the risk of atrial fibrillation was lower (hazard ratio, 0.79; 95 percent confidence interval, 0.66 to 0.94; P=0.008), and heart-failure scores were better (P<0.001). The differences in the rates of hospitalization for heart failure and of death, stroke, or hospitalization for heart failure were not significant in unadjusted analyses but became marginally significant in adjusted analyses. Dual-chamber pacing resulted in a small but measurable increase in the quality of life, as compared with ventricular pacing.

CONCLUSIONS

In sinus-node dysfunction, dual-chamber pacing does not improve stroke-free survival, as compared with ventricular pacing. However, dual-chamber pacing reduces the risk of atrial fibrillation, reduces signs and symptoms of heart failure, and slightly improves the quality of life. Overall, dual-chamber pacing offers significant improvement as compared with ventricular pacing.

DAVID TRIAL
THE DUAL CHAMBER AND VVI IMPLANTABLE DEFIBRILLATOR (DAVID) TRIAL: RATIONALE, DESIGN, RESULTS, CLINICAL IMPLICATIONS AND LESSONS FOR FUTURE TRIALS.
CARDIAC ELECTROPHYSIOLOGY REVIEW 2003.

In DAVID trail patients with heart failure and indication for ICD implant were randomized into two groups, first with dual-chamber pacing mode, and the second group with only back-up pacing mode. With the hypothesis that dual-chamber pacing will improve hemodynamic in these patients. What was found that high percentage of RV pacing (in the absence of pacing indications) lead to a worse outcome than patients with ICDs programmed to only backup pacing. The RV pacing-induced dyssynchrony had deleterious effects. It was concluded that patients with indications for implantable defibrillators and no indication for pacing should not be paced in the dual chamber pacing mode.

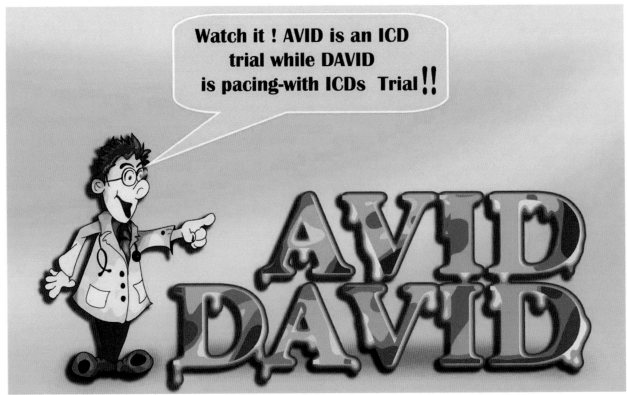

DAVID TRIAL

The Dual Chamber and VVI Implantable Defibrillator (DAVID) Trial: rationale, design, results, clinical implications and lessons for future trials.

Wilkoff BL; et al.

Cardiac electrophysiology review 2003; December7; (4):468-72.

T he Dual Chamber and VVI Implantable Defibrillator (DAVID) trial randomized 506 patients and tested the hypothesis that the dual-chamber pacing mode would produce improved hemodynamics and would in turn reduce congestive heart failure, heart failure hospitalizations, heart failure deaths, atrial fibrillation, strokes, ventricular arrhythmias, and total mortality compared to backup ventricular pacing in patients indicated for implantable defibrillator therapy. Patients had either primary prevention indications (47%) or secondary prevention indications (53%) for implantable defibrillator therapy but had no indications for bradycardia pacemaker support. All the patients had moderate to severe left ventricular dysfunction with a left ventricular ejection fraction of 40% or less (mean = 27%) and were consistently treated with angiotensin converting enzyme inhibitors or angiotensin II receptor blockers (86%) and beta adrenergic blocking agents (85%). The primary combined endpoint of hospitalization for congestive heart failure or death was paradoxically increased and statistically significant ($p = 0.03$) at one year in the patients paced in the dual chamber mode (22.6%) compared to patients randomized to ventricular backup pacing (13.3%). Both heart failure hospitalization and mortality contributed outcome. Another perspective would consider this a randomized controlled study of presence or absence of pacemaker therapy in patients with left ventricular dysfunction and indications for implantable defibrillator therapy. Ventricular backup pacing produced less than 3% ventricular and no atrial pacing, while dual chamber pacing produced approximately 60% atrial and ventricular paced heart beats. The poor outcome in the dual chamber paced group correlated with the percentage of right ventricular pacing and suggests that right ventricular pacing caused ventricular dyssynchrony. The poor outcome associated with right ventricular pacing compared to intrinsic activation in the control group of the DAVID trial is reminiscent of the poor outcome associated with prolonged intraventricular conduction activation in the control groups compared to biventricular pacing in the intervention groups of the cardiac resynchronization trials. The direct conclusion from these results are that patients with indications for implantable defibrillators and no indication for pacing should not be paced in the dual chamber pacing mode. It is not appropriate to conclude that only single chamber implantable defibrillators should be implanted. There are other potential advantages to having an implanted atrial lead including improved secondary outcomes. However the DAVID trial results suggest that the dual chamber paced mode was not associated with improved quality of life or decreased frequency of hospitalization, inappropriate shocks from the defibrillator or atrial fibrillation. The more important question is what is the optimal pacing mode in these patients? The AAIR mode is under investigation in the DAVID II study in an attempt to identify a pacing mode that preserves atrio-ventricular synchrony, normal atrio-ventricular timing, prevents bradycardia and also prevents right ventricular stimulation. Caution should be taken to not directly apply these results to patients with either an indication for pacemaker therapy or to patients with an indication for cardiac resynchronization therapy since patients from neither population were included. However, considering the large magnitude of the deleterious effects associated with dual chamber pacing in the DAVID trial future studies should explore the possibility that left ventricular stimulation may be the only pacing mode capable of preventing bradycardia without increasing death and congestive heart failure.

Miscellaneous Trials
"HTN, HLP, others"

WEST OF SCOTLAND CORONARY PREVENTION STUDY(WOSCOPS)
WEST OF SCOTLAND CORONARY PREVENTION STUDY: IDENTIFICATION OF HIGH-RISK GROUPS AND COMPARISON WITH OTHER CARDIOVASCULAR INTERVENTION TRIALS.
LANCET. 1996.

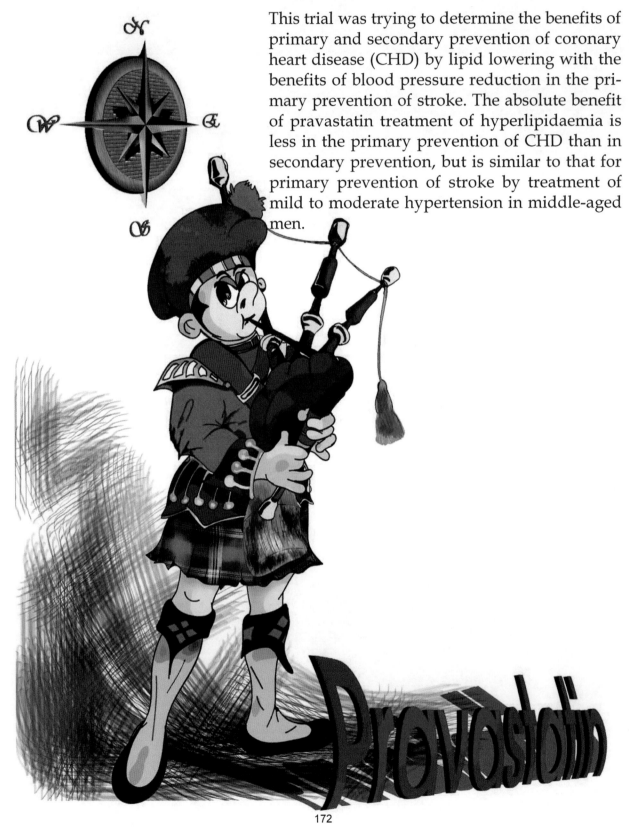

This trial was trying to determine the benefits of primary and secondary prevention of coronary heart disease (CHD) by lipid lowering with the benefits of blood pressure reduction in the primary prevention of stroke. The absolute benefit of pravastatin treatment of hyperlipidaemia is less in the primary prevention of CHD than in secondary prevention, but is similar to that for primary prevention of stroke by treatment of mild to moderate hypertension in middle-aged men.

West of Scotland Coronary Prevention Study (WOSCOPS)
West of Scotland Coronary Prevention Study: identification of high-risk groups and comparison with other cardiovascular intervention trials.

Lancet. 1996; November; 16;348(9038):1339-42.

BACKGROUND

We assessed the potential benefit of treatment for low-risk and high-risk groups in the West of Scotland Coronary Prevention Study (WOSCOPS) population, and compared the benefits of primary and secondary prevention of coronary heart disease (CHD) by lipid lowering with the benefits of blood pressure reduction in the primary prevention of stroke.

METHODS

We did a subgroup analysis of placebo-treated men in the WOSCOPS population by age, vascular disease at trial entry, and other established risk factors. We also compared WOSCOPS findings with those of the Scandinavian Simvastatin Survival Study (4S) and the Medical Research Council (MRC) trial of treatment for mild to moderate hypertension in middle-aged men. The WOSCOPS population comprised 6595 men aged 45-64 years with no history of myocardial infarction (MI) and plasma total cholesterol concentrations of 6.5-8.0 mmol/L at initial screening. Participants were randomly allocated pravastatin (40 mg daily) or placebo, and followed up for an average of 4.9 years.

FINDINGS

Coronary event rates at 5 years in the WOSCOPS placebo group were higher than 10% (the recommended treatment threshold) in men with pre-existing vascular disease and in those 55 years or older without symptoms or signs of CHD but with at least one other risk factor. Event rates were low in men with hypercholesterolaemia but no other risk factor: 3.5% (95% CI 1.3-5.7) for men aged 45-54 years and 5.3% (2.7-8.0) for men aged 55-64 years. Three times more men had to be treated for 5 years to prevent one endpoint in WOSCOPS than in 4S. By contrast, two to four times fewer men with hyperlipidaemia were treated to save one coronary event in WOSCOPS than hypertensives to save one stroke in the MRC trial. These differences persisted after adjustment for the low-risk status of many of the patients with hypertension who took part in the MRC trial.

INTERPRETATION

There were a substantial number of men whose risk of a coronary event was more than 10% at 5 years in the WOSCOPS cohort. The absolute benefit of pravastatin treatment of hyperlipidaemia is less in the primary prevention of CHD than in secondary prevention, but is similar to that for primary prevention of stroke by treatment of mild to moderate hypertension in middle-aged men.

HEART PROTECTION STUDY

MRC/BHF HEART PROTECTION STUDY OF CHOLESTEROL LOWERING WITH SIMVASTATIN IN 20,536 HIGH-RISK INDIVIDUALS: A RANDOMISED PLACEBO-CONTROLLED TRIAL.

LANCET. 2002

This trial was trying to determine whether reducing LDL cholesterol irrespective of initial cholesterol concentrations may reduce the development of vascular disease. Results showed that adding 40 mg of simvastatin (compared to placebo) to existing treatments safely produces substantial additional benefits for a wide range of high-risk patients, irrespective of their initial cholesterol concentrations. A significant reduction in the rates of myocardial infarction, of stroke, and of revascularization was noted in treatment group.

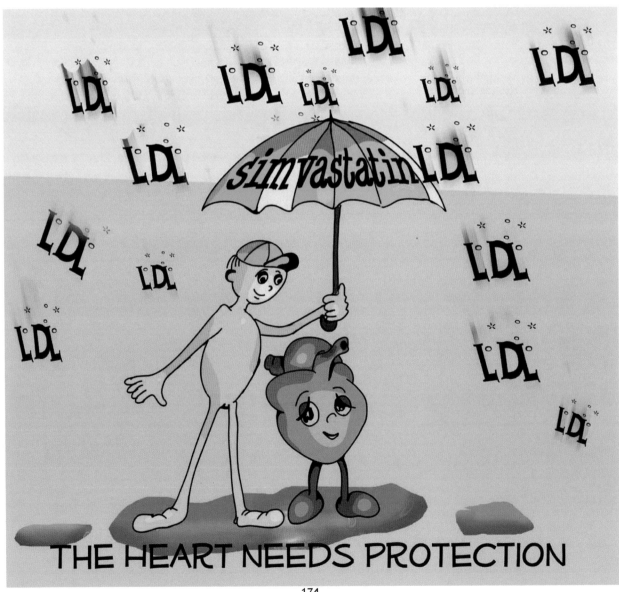

Heart Protection Study

MRC/BHF Heart Protection Study of cholesterol lowering with simvastatin in 20,536 high-risk individuals: a randomised placebo-controlled trial.

Heart Protection Study Collaborative Group.

Lancet. 2002 July 6;360(9326):7-22.

BACKGROUND

Throughout the usual LDL cholesterol range in Western populations, lower blood concentrations are associated with lower cardiovascular disease risk. In such populations, therefore, reducing LDL cholesterol may reduce the development of vascular disease, largely irrespective of initial cholesterol concentrations.

METHODS

20,536 UK adults (aged 40-80 years) with coronary disease, other occlusive arterial disease, or diabetes were randomly allocated to receive 40 mg simvastatin daily (average compliance: 85%) or matching placebo (average non-study statin use: 17%). Analyses are of the first occurrence of particular events, and compare all simvastatin-allocated versus all placebo-allocated participants. These "intention-to-treat" comparisons assess the effects of about two-thirds (85% minus 17%) taking a statin during the scheduled 5-year treatment period, which yielded an average difference in LDL cholesterol of 1.0 mmol/L (about two-thirds of the effect of actual use of 40 mg simvastatin daily). Primary outcomes were mortality (for overall analyses) and fatal or non-fatal vascular events (for subcategory analyses), with subsidiary assessments of cancer and of other major morbidity.

FINDINGS

All-cause mortality was significantly reduced (1328 [12.9%] deaths among 10,269 allocated simvastatin versus 1507 [14.7%] among 10,267 allocated placebo; p=0.0003), due to a highly significant 18% (SE 5) proportional reduction in the coronary death rate (587 [5.7%] vs 707 [6.9%]; p=0.0005), a marginally significant reduction in other vascular deaths (194 [1.9%] vs 230 [2.2%]; p=0.07), and a non-significant reduction in non-vascular deaths (547 [5.3%] vs 570 [5.6%]; p=0.4). There were highly significant reductions of about one-quarter in the first event rate for non-fatal myocardial infarction or coronary death (898 [8.7%] vs 1212 [11.8%]; p<0.0001), for non-fatal or fatal stroke (444 [4.3%] vs 585 [5.7%]; p<0.0001), and for coronary or non-coronary revascularisation (939 [9.1%] vs 1205 [11.7%]; p<0.0001). For the first occurrence of any of these major vascular events, there was a definite 24% (SE 3; 95% CI 19-28) reduction in the event rate (2033 [19.8%] vs 2585 [25.2%] affected individuals; p<0.0001). During the first year the reduction in major vascular events was not significant, but subsequently it was highly significant during each separate year. The proportional reduction in the event rate was similar (and significant) in each subcategory of participant studied, including: those without diagnosed coronary disease who had cerebrovascular disease, or had peripheral artery disease, or had diabetes; men and, separately, women; those aged either under or over 70 years at entry; and--most notably--even those who presented with LDL cholesterol below 3.0 mmol/L (116 mg/dL), or total cholesterol below 5.0 mmol/L (193 mg/dL). The benefits of simvastatin were additional to those of other cardioprotective treatments. The annual excess risk of myopathy with this regimen was about 0.01%. There were no significant adverse effects on cancer incidence or on hospitalisation for any other non-vascular cause.

INTERPRETATION

Adding simvastatin to existing treatments safely produces substantial additional benefits for a wide range of high-risk patients, irrespective of their initial cholesterol concentrations. Allocation to 40 mg simvastatin daily reduced the rates of myocardial infarction, of stroke, and of revascularisation by about one-quarter. After making allowance for non-compliance, actual use of this regimen would probably reduce these rates by about one-third. Hence, among the many types of high-risk individual studied, 5 years of simvastatin would prevent about 70-100 people per 1000 from suffering at least one of these major vascular events (and longer treatment should produce further benefit). The size of the 5-year benefit depends chiefly on such individuals' overall risk of major vascular events, rather than on their blood lipid concentrations alone

JUPITER TRIAL
ROSUVASTATIN TO PREVENT VASCULAR EVENTS IN MEN AND WOMEN WITH ELEVATED C-REACTIVE PROTEIN.
NEW ENGLAND JOURNAL OF MEDICINE (NEJM) 2008.

This trial was trying to determine whether people with elevated high-sensitivity C-reactive protein, which is a marker that predicts cardiovascular events, might benefit from statin treatment even if they don't have hyperlipidemia. Since statin therapy is known to have anti-inflammatory effects. Results showed that among apparently healthy individuals without hyperlipidemia but with elevated high-sensitivity C-reactive protein levels, rosuvastatin significantly reduced the incidence of major cardiovascular events.

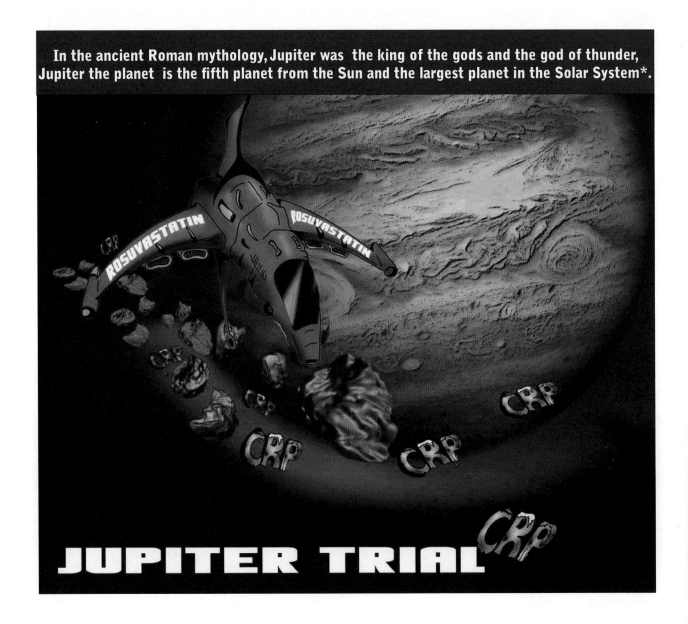

In the ancient Roman mythology, Jupiter was the king of the gods and the god of thunder, Jupiter the planet is the fifth planet from the Sun and the largest planet in the Solar System*.

JUPITER TRIAL

*http://en.wikipedia.org

JUPITER TRIAL

Rosuvastatin to prevent vascular events in men and women with elevated C-reactive protein.

Ridker PM, et al. JUPITER Study Group.

New England Journal of Medicine (NEJM) 2008; November 20; 359(21):2195-207.

BACKGROUND:

Increased levels of the inflammatory biomarker high-sensitivity C-reactive protein predict cardiovascular events. Since statins lower levels of high-sensitivity C-reactive protein as well as cholesterol, we hypothesized that people with elevated high-sensitivity C-reactive protein levels but without hyperlipidemia might benefit from statin treatment.

METHODS:

We randomly assigned 17,802 apparently healthy men and women with low-density lipoprotein (LDL) cholesterol levels of less than 130 mg per deciliter (3.4 mmol per liter) and high-sensitivity C-reactive protein levels of 2.0 mg per liter or higher to rosuvastatin, 20 mg daily, or placebo and followed them for the occurrence of the combined primary end point of myocardial infarction, stroke, arterial revascularization, hospitalization for unstable angina, or death from cardiovascular causes.

RESULTS:

The trial was stopped after a median follow-up of 1.9 years (maximum, 5.0). Rosuvastatin reduced LDL cholesterol levels by 50% and high-sensitivity C-reactive protein levels by 37%. The rates of the primary end point were 0.77 and 1.36 per 100 person-years of follow-up in the rosuvastatin and placebo groups, respectively (hazard ratio for rosuvastatin, 0.56; 95% confidence interval [CI], 0.46 to 0.69; $P<0.00001$), with corresponding rates of 0.17 and 0.37 for myocardial infarction (hazard ratio, 0.46; 95% CI, 0.30 to 0.70; $P=0.0002$), 0.18 and 0.34 for stroke (hazard ratio, 0.52; 95% CI, 0.34 to 0.79; $P=0.002$), 0.41 and 0.77 for revascularization or unstable angina (hazard ratio, 0.53; 95% CI, 0.40 to 0.70; $P<0.00001$), 0.45 and 0.85 for the combined end point of myocardial infarction, stroke, or death from cardiovascular causes (hazard ratio, 0.53; 95% CI, 0.40 to 0.69; $P<0.00001$), and 1.00 and 1.25 for death from any cause (hazard ratio, 0.80; 95% CI, 0.67 to 0.97; $P=0.02$). Consistent effects were observed in all subgroups evaluated. The rosuvastatin group did not have a significant increase in myopathy or cancer but did have a higher incidence of physician-reported diabetes.

CONCLUSIONS:

In this trial of apparently healthy persons without hyperlipidemia but with elevated high-sensitivity C-reactive protein levels, rosuvastatin significantly reduced the incidence of major cardiovascular events.

ASTEROID TRIAL

EFFECT OF VERY HIGH-INTENSITY STATIN THERAPY ON REGRESSION OF CORONARY ATHEROSCLEROSIS: THE ASTEROID TRIAL. NISSEN SE, ET AL. ASTEROID INVESTIGATORS.
JOURNAL OF THE AMERICAN MEDICAL ASSOCIATION (JAMA) 2006; APRIL 5; 295(13):1556-65.

ASTEROID trial was the first trial to show significant regression of atherosclerosis determined by Intravascular ultrasound (IVUS), using high-intensity statin therapy using rosuvastatin 40 mg.

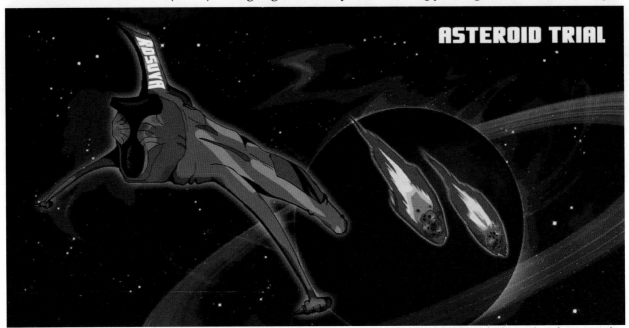

CONTEXT: Prior intravascular ultrasound (IVUS) trials have demonstrated slowing or halting of atherosclerosis progression with statin therapy but have not shown convincing evidence of regression using percent atheroma volume (PAV), the most rigorous IVUS measure of disease progression and regression.

OBJECTIVE: To assess whether very intensive statin therapy could regress coronary atherosclerosis as determined by IVUS imaging.

DESIGN AND SETTING: Prospective, open-label blinded end-points trial (A Study to Evaluate the Effect of Rosuvastatin on Intravascular Ultrasound-Derived Coronary Atheroma Burden [ASTEROID]) was performed at 53 community and tertiary care centers in the United States, Canada, Europe, and Australia. A motorized IVUS pullback was used to assess coronary atheroma burden at baseline and after 24 months of treatment. Each pair of baseline and follow-up IVUS assessments was analyzed in a blinded fashion.

PATIENTS: Between November 2002 and October 2003, 507 patients had a baseline IVUS examination and received at least 1 dose of study drug. After 24 months, 349 patients had evaluable serial IVUS examinations.

INTERVENTION: All patients received intensive statin therapy with rosuvastatin, 40 mg/d.

MAIN OUTCOME MEASURES: Two primary efficacy parameters were prespecified: the change in PAV and the change in nominal atheroma volume in the 10-mm subsegment with the greatest disease severity at baseline. A secondary efficacy variable, change in normalized total atheroma volume for the entire artery, was also prespecified.

RESULTS: The mean (SD) baseline low-density lipoprotein cholesterol (LDL-C) level of 130.4 (34.3) mg/dL declined to 60.8 (20.0) mg/dL, a mean reduction of 53.2% (P<.001). Mean (SD) high-density lipoprotein cholesterol (HDL-C) level at baseline was 43.1 (11.1) mg/dL, increasing to 49.0 (12.6) mg/dL, an increase of 14.7% (P<.001). The mean (SD) change in PAV for the entire vessel was -0.98% (3.15%), with a median of -0.79% (97.5% CI, -1.21% to -0.53%) (P<.001 vs baseline). The mean (SD) change in atheroma volume in the most diseased 10-mm subsegment was -6.1 (10.1) mm3, with a median of -5.6 mm3 (97.5% CI, -6.8 to -4.0 mm3) (P<.001 vs baseline). Change in total atheroma volume showed a 6.8% median reduction; with a mean (SD) reduction of -14.7 (25.7) mm3, with a median of -12.5 mm3 (95% CI, -15.1 to -10.5 mm3) (P<.001 vs baseline). Adverse events were infrequent and similar to other statin trials.

CONCLUSIONS: Very high-intensity statin therapy using rosuvastatin 40 mg/d achieved an average LDL-C of 60.8 mg/dL and increased HDL-C by 14.7%, resulting in significant regression of atherosclerosis for all 3 prespecified IVUS measures of disease burden. Treatment to LDL-C levels below currently accepted guidelines, when accompanied by significant HDL-C increases, can regress atherosclerosis in coronary disease patients. Further studies are needed to determine the effect of the observed changes on clinical outcome.

4S TRIAL

Randomised trial of cholesterol lowering in 4444 patients with coronary heart disease: the Scandinavian Simvastatin Survival Study (4S)
Lancet. 1994 November 19;344(8934):1383-9.

Drug therapy for hypercholesterolaemia has remained controversial mainly because of insufficient clinical trial evidence for improved survival. The present trial was designed to evaluate the effect of cholesterol lowering with simvastatin on mortality and morbidity in patients with coronary heart disease (CHD). 4444 patients with angina pectoris or previous myocardial infarction and serum cholesterol 5.5-8.0 mmol/L on a lipid-lowering diet were randomised to double-blind treatment with simvastatin or placebo. Over the 5.4 years median follow-up period, simvastatin produced mean changes in total cholesterol, low-density-lipoprotein cholesterol, and high-density-lipoprotein cholesterol of -25%, -35%, and +8%, respectively, with few adverse effects. 256 patients (12%) in the placebo group died, compared with 182 (8%) in the simvastatin group. The relative risk of death in the simvastatin group was 0.70 (95% CI 0.58-0.85, p = 0.0003). The 6-year probabilities of survival in the placebo and simvastatin groups were 87.6% and 91.3%, respectively. There were 189 coronary deaths in the placebo group and 111 in the simvastatin group (relative risk 0.58, 95% CI 0.46-0.73), while noncardiovascular causes accounted for 49 and 46 deaths, respectively. 622 patients (28%) in the placebo group and 431 (19%) in the simvastatin group had one or more major coronary events. The relative risk was 0.66 (95% CI 0.59-0.75, p < 0.00001), and the respective probabilities of escaping such events were 70.5% and 79.6%. This risk was also significantly reduced in subgroups consisting of women and patients of both sexes aged 60 or more. Other benefits of treatment included a 37% reduction (p < 0.00001) in the risk of undergoing myocardial revascularisation procedures. This study shows that long-term treatment with simvastatin is safe and improves survival in CHD patients.

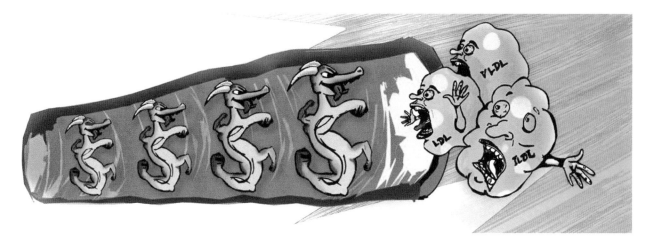

4S TRIAL

This trial was the first trial trying to evaluate the effect of cholesterol lowering (with simvastatin) on mortality and morbidity in patients with coronary heart disease (CHD). Results showed that that long-term treatment with simvastatin is safe and improves survival in CHD patients.

TNT TRIAL

INTENSIVE LIPID LOWERING WITH ATORVASTATIN IN PATIENTS WITH STABLE CORONARY DISEASE.
LAROSA JC, ET AL. TREATING TO NEW TARGETS (TNT) INVESTIGATORS.
NEW ENGLAND JOURNAL OF MEDICINE (NEJM) 2005.

This trial was trying to determine the efficacy and safety of lowering LDL cholesterol levels below 100 mg per deciliter in patients with stable coronary heart disease (CHD) using 80 mg of atorvastatin vs. 10 mg of atorvastatin daily. The 80 mg daily showed significant reduction of the primary end point (occurrence of a first major cardiovascular event, defined as death from CHD, nonfatal non-procedure-related myocardial infarction, resuscitation after cardiac arrest, or fatal or nonfatal stroke) with only a slight increase in the aminotransferase levels.

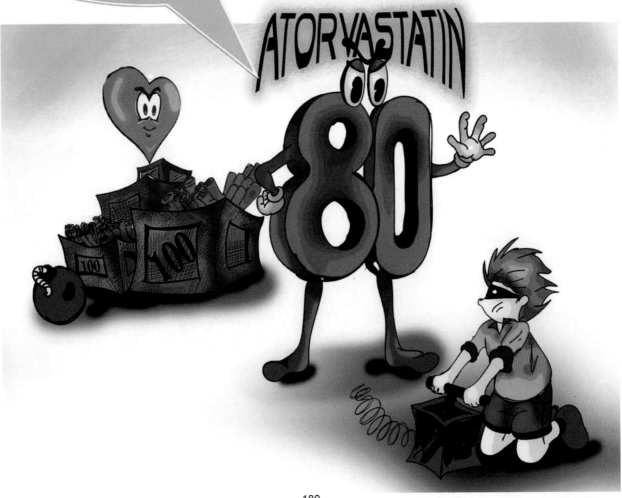

TNT TRIAL
Intensive lipid lowering with atorvastatin in patients with stable coronary disease.
LaRosa JC, et al. Treating to New Targets (TNT) Investigators.
New England Journal of Medicine (NEJM) 2005; April; 7;352(14):1425-35.

BACKGROUND
Previous trials have demonstrated that lowering low-density lipoprotein (LDL) cholesterol levels below currently recommended levels is beneficial in patients with acute coronary syndromes. We prospectively assessed the efficacy and safety of lowering LDL cholesterol levels below 100 mg per deciliter (2.6 mmol per liter) in patients with stable coronary heart disease (CHD).

METHODS
A total of 10,001 patients with clinically evident CHD and LDL cholesterol levels of less than 130 mg per deciliter (3.4 mmol per liter) were randomly assigned to double-blind therapy and received either 10 mg or 80 mg of atorvastatin per day. Patients were followed for a median of 4.9 years. The primary end point was the occurrence of a first major cardiovascular event, defined as death from CHD, nonfatal non-procedure-related myocardial infarction, resuscitation after cardiac arrest, or fatal or nonfatal stroke.

RESULTS
The mean LDL cholesterol levels were 77 mg per deciliter (2.0 mmol per liter) during treatment with 80 mg of atorvastatin and 101 mg per deciliter (2.6 mmol per liter) during treatment with 10 mg of atorvastatin. The incidence of persistent elevations in liver aminotransferase levels was 0.2 percent in the group given 10 mg of atorvastatin and 1.2 percent in the group given 80 mg of atorvastatin (P<0.001). A primary event occurred in 434 patients (8.7 percent) receiving 80 mg of atorvastatin, as compared with 548 patients (10.9 percent) receiving 10 mg of atorvastatin, representing an absolute reduction in the rate of major cardiovascular events of 2.2 percent and a 22 percent relative reduction in risk (hazard ratio, 0.78; 95 percent confidence interval, 0.69 to 0.89; P<0.001). There was no difference between the two treatment groups in overall mortality.

CONCLUSIONS
Intensive lipid-lowering therapy with 80 mg of atorvastatin per day in patients with stable CHD provides significant clinical benefit beyond that afforded by treatment with 10 mg of atorvastatin per day. This occurred with a greater incidence of elevated aminotransferase levels.

PEACE AND EUROPEAN TRIALS

Both of these trials tested the potential benefit of ACE-inhibitors in patients with stable coronary artery disease without LV dysfunction. PEACE trial did not show any reduction in cardiovascular events with treatment with trandolapril versus placebo. On the other hand the EURopean trial used Perindopril in similar set of patients and showed an improved outcome, although it seemed that 50 patients need to be treated for a period of 4 years to prevent one major cardiovascular event.

Some people believe in HIPPIES some people don't.. Some trials say ACE-I is good regardless of your EF some trials say they are not !

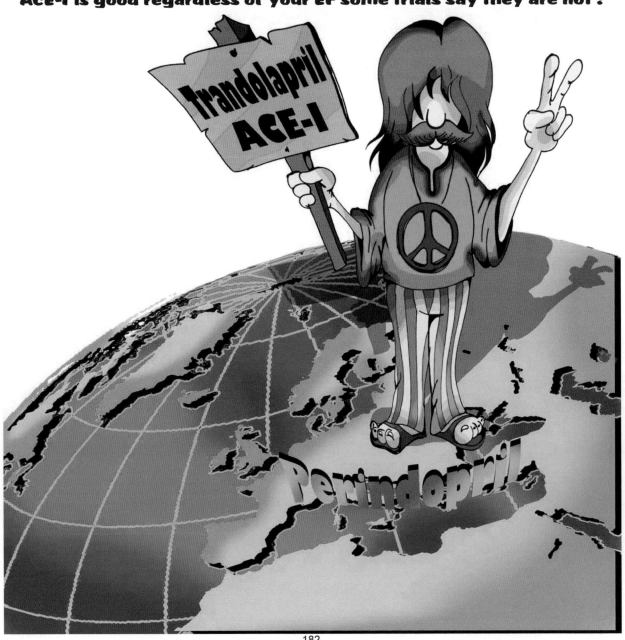

PEACE Trial

Angiotensin-converting-enzyme inhibition in stable coronary artery disease.

Braunwald E et al.

New England Journal of Medicine (NEJM) 2004; November 11;351(20):2058-68.

BACKGROUND

Angiotensin-converting-enzyme (ACE) inhibitors are effective in reducing the risk of heart failure, myocardial infarction, and death from cardiovascular causes in patients with left ventricular systolic dysfunction or heart failure. ACE inhibitors have also been shown to reduce atherosclerotic complications in patients who have vascular disease without heart failure.

METHODS

In the Prevention of Events with Angiotensin Converting Enzyme Inhibition (PEACE) Trial, we tested the hypothesis that patients with stable coronary artery disease and normal or slightly reduced left ventricular function derive therapeutic benefit from the addition of ACE inhibitors to modern conventional therapy. The trial was a double-blind, placebo-controlled study in which 8290 patients were randomly assigned to receive either trandolapril at a target dose of 4 mg per day (4158 patients) or matching placebo (4132 patients).

RESULTS

The mean (+/-SD) age of the patients was 64+/-8 years, the mean blood pressure 133+/-17/78+/-10 mm Hg, and the mean left ventricular ejection fraction 58+/-9 percent. The patients received intensive treatment, with 72 percent having previously undergone coronary revascularization and 70 percent receiving lipid-lowering drugs. The incidence of the primary end point--death from cardiovascular causes, myocardial infarction, or coronary revascularization--was 21.9 percent in the trandolapril group, as compared with 22.5 percent in the placebo group (hazard ratio in the trandolapril group, 0.96; 95 percent confidence interval, 0.88 to 1.06; P=0.43) over a median follow-up period of 4.8 years.

CONCLUSIONS

In patients with stable coronary heart disease and preserved left ventricular function who are receiving "current standard" therapy and in whom the rate of cardiovascular events is lower than in previous trials of ACE inhibitors in patients with vascular disease, there is no evidence that the addition of an ACE inhibitor provides further benefit in terms of death from cardiovascular causes, myocardial infarction, or coronary revascularization.

EURopean trial

Efficacy of perindopril in reduction of cardiovascular events among patients with stable coronary artery disease: randomised, double-blind, placebo-controlled, multi-centre trial (the EUROPA study). Fox KM et al.

Lancet. 2003 September 6;362(9386):782-8.

BACKGROUND

Treatment with angiotensin-converting-enzyme (ACE) inhibitors reduces the rate of cardiovascular events among patients with left-ventricular dysfunction and those at high risk of such events. We assessed whether the ACE inhibitor perindopril reduced cardiovascular risk in a low-risk population with stable coronary heart disease and no apparent heart failure.

METHODS

We recruited patients from October, 1997, to June, 2000. 13655 patients were registered with previous myocardial infarction (64%), angiographic evidence of coronary artery disease (61%), coronary revascularisation (55%), or a positive stress test only (5%). After a run-in period of 4 weeks, in which all patients received perindopril, 12218 patients were randomly assigned perindopril 8 mg once daily (n=6110), or matching placebo (n=6108). The mean follow-up was 4.2 years, and the primary endpoint was cardiovascular death, myocardial infarction, or cardiac arrest. Analysis was by intention to treat.

FINDINGS

Mean age of patients was 60 years (SD 9), 85% were male, 92% were taking platelet inhibitors, 62% beta blockers, and 58% lipid-lowering therapy. 603 (10%) placebo and 488 (8%) perindopril patients experienced the primary endpoint, which yields a 20% relative risk reduction (95% CI 9-29, p=0.0003) with perindopril. These benefits were consistent in all predefined subgroups and secondary endpoints. Perindopril was well tolerated.

INTERPRETATION

Among patients with stable coronary heart disease without apparent heart failure, perindopril can significantly improve outcome. About 50 patients need to be treated for a period of 4 years to prevent one major cardiovascular event. Treatment with perindopril, on top of other preventive medications, should be considered in all patients with coronary heart disease.

ALLHAT TRIAL

MAJOR OUTCOMES IN HIGH-RISK HYPERTENSIVE PATIENTS RANDOMIZED TO ANGIOTENSIN-CONVERTING ENZYME INHIBITOR OR CALCIUM CHANNEL BLOCKER VS DIURETIC: THE ANTIHYPERTENSIVE AND LIPID-LOWERING TREATMENT TO PREVENT HEART ATTACK TRIAL (ALLHAT).
JOURNAL OF THE AMERICAN MEDICAL ASSOCIATION (JAMA). 2002 .

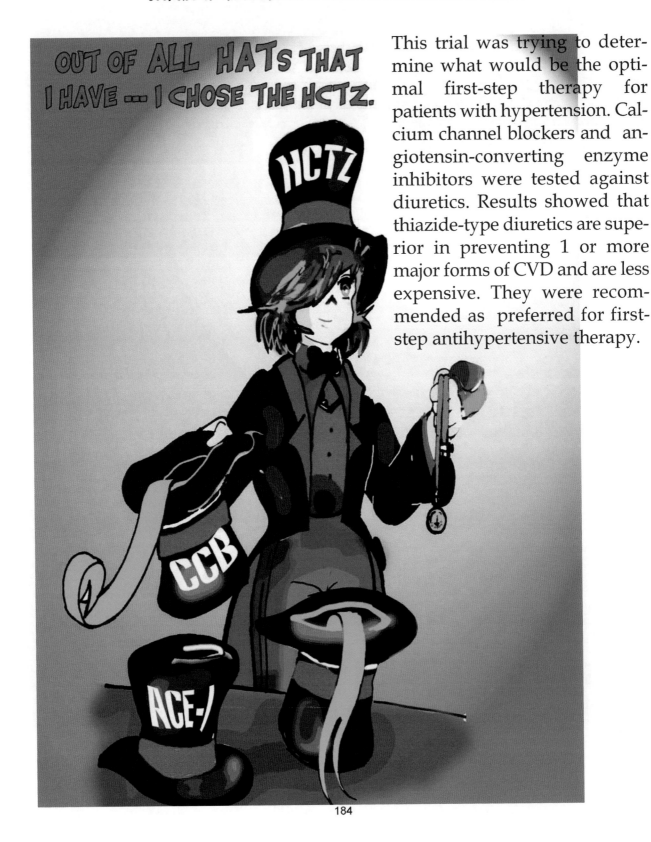

This trial was trying to determine what would be the optimal first-step therapy for patients with hypertension. Calcium channel blockers and angiotensin-converting enzyme inhibitors were tested against diuretics. Results showed that thiazide-type diuretics are superior in preventing 1 or more major forms of CVD and are less expensive. They were recommended as preferred for first-step antihypertensive therapy.

ALLHAT TRIAL

Major outcomes in high-risk hypertensive patients randomized to angiotensin-converting enzyme inhibitor or calcium channel blocker vs diuretic: The Antihypertensive and Lipid-Lowering Treatment to Prevent Heart Attack Trial (ALLHAT).
ALLHAT Officers and Coordinators for the ALLHAT Collaborative Research Group. The Antihypertensive and Lipid-Lowering Treatment to Prevent Heart Attack Trial.

Journal of the American Medical Association (JAMA). 2002 December 18;288(23):2981-97.

CONTEXT:

Antihypertensive therapy is well established to reduce hypertension-related morbidity and mortality, but the optimal first-step therapy is unknown.

OBJECTIVE:

To determine whether treatment with a calcium channel blocker or an angiotensin-converting enzyme inhibitor lowers the incidence of coronary heart disease (CHD) or other cardiovascular disease (CVD) events vs treatment with a diuretic.

DESIGN:

The Antihypertensive and Lipid-Lowering Treatment to Prevent Heart Attack Trial (ALLHAT), a randomized, double-blind, active-controlled clinical trial conducted from February 1994 through March 2002.

SETTING AND PARTICIPANTS:

A total of 33 357 participants aged 55 years or older with hypertension and at least 1 other CHD risk factor from 623 North American centers.

INTERVENTIONS:

Participants were randomly assigned to receive chlorthalidone, 12.5 to 25 mg/d (n = 15 255); amlodipine, 2.5 to 10 mg/d (n = 9048); or lisinopril, 10 to 40 mg/d (n = 9054) for planned follow-up of approximately 4 to 8 years.

MAIN OUTCOME MEASURES:

The primary outcome was combined fatal CHD or nonfatal myocardial infarction, analyzed by intent-to-treat. Secondary outcomes were all-cause mortality, stroke, combined CHD (primary outcome, coronary revascularization, or angina with hospitalization), and combined CVD (combined CHD, stroke, treated angina without hospitalization, heart failure [HF], and peripheral arterial disease).

RESULTS:

Mean follow-up was 4.9 years. The primary outcome occurred in 2956 participants, with no difference between treatments. Compared with chlorthalidone (6-year rate, 11.5%), the relative risks (RRs) were 0.98 (95% CI, 0.90-1.07) for amlodipine (6-year rate, 11.3%) and 0.99 (95% CI, 0.91-1.08) for lisinopril (6-year rate, 11.4%). Likewise, all-cause mortality did not differ between groups. Five-year systolic blood pressures were significantly higher in the amlodipine (0.8 mm Hg, P =.03) and lisinopril (2 mm Hg, P<.001) groups compared with chlorthalidone, and 5-year diastolic blood pressure was significantly lower with amlodipine (0.8 mm Hg, P<.001). For amlodipine vs chlorthalidone, secondary outcomes were similar except for a higher 6-year rate of HF with amlodipine (10.2% vs 7.7%; RR, 1.38; 95% CI, 1.25-1.52). For lisinopril vs chlorthalidone, lisinopril had higher 6-year rates of combined CVD (33.3% vs 30.9%; RR, 1.10; 95% CI, 1.05-1.16); stroke (6.3% vs 5.6%; RR, 1.15; 95% CI, 1.02-1.30); and HF (8.7% vs 7.7%; RR, 1.19; 95% CI, 1.07-1.31).

CONCLUSION:

Thiazide-type diuretics are superior in preventing 1 or more major forms of CVD and are less expensive. They should be preferred for first-step antihypertensive therapy.

HOPE TRIAL

EFFECTS OF AN ANGIOTENSIN-CONVERTING-ENZYME INHIBITOR, RAMIPRIL, ON CARDIOVASCULAR EVENTS IN HIGH-RISK PATIENTS.

NEW ENGLAND JOURNAL OF MEDICINE (NEJM) 2000.

This trial was trying to assess the role of an angiotensin-converting-enzyme inhibitor, ramipril, in patients who were at high risk for cardiovascular events but who did not have left ventricular dysfunction or heart failure. Results showed that Ramipril significantly reduces the rates of death, myocardial infarction, and stroke in a broad range of high-risk patients who are not known to have a low ejection fraction or heart failure.

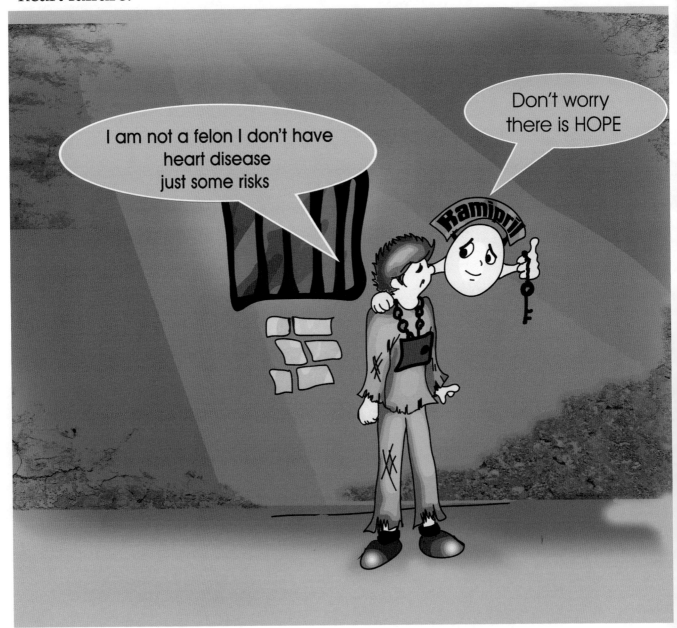

HOPE TRIAL

Effects of an angiotensin-converting-enzyme inhibitor, ramipril, on cardiovascular events in high-risk patients. The Heart Outcomes Prevention Evaluation Study Investigators. Yusuf S et al.

New England Journal of Medicine (NEJM) 2000 January 20;342(3):145-53.

BACKGROUND:

Angiotensin-converting-enzyme inhibitors improve the outcome among patients with left ventricular dysfunction, whether or not they have heart failure. We assessed the role of an angiotensin-converting-enzyme inhibitor, ramipril, in patients who were at high risk for cardiovascular events but who did not have left ventricular dysfunction or heart failure.

METHODS:

A total of 9297 high-risk patients (55 years of age or older) who had evidence of vascular disease or diabetes plus one other cardiovascular risk factor and who were not known to have a low ejection fraction or heart failure were randomly assigned to receive ramipril (10 mg once per day orally) or matching placebo for a mean of five years. The primary outcome was a composite of myocardial infarction, stroke, or death from cardiovascular causes. The trial was a two-by-two factorial study evaluating both ramipril and vitamin E. The effects of vitamin E are reported in a companion paper.

RESULTS:

A total of 651 patients who were assigned to receive ramipril (14.0 percent) reached the primary end point, as compared with 826 patients who were assigned to receive placebo (17.8 percent) (relative risk, 0.78; 95 percent confidence interval, 0.70 to 0.86; P<0.001). Treatment with ramipril reduced the rates of death from cardiovascular causes (6.1 percent, as compared with 8.1 percent in the placebo group; relative risk, 0.74; P<0.001), myocardial infarction (9.9 percent vs. 12.3 percent; relative risk, 0.80; P<0.001), stroke (3.4 percent vs. 4.9 percent; relative risk, 0.68; P<0.001), death from any cause (10.4 percent vs. 12.2 percent; relative risk, 0.84; P=0.005), revascularization procedures (16.3 percent vs. 18.8 percent; relative risk, 0.85; P<0.001), cardiac arrest (0.8 percent vs. 1.3 percent; relative risk, 0.62; P=0.02), [corrected] heart failure (9.1 percent vs. 11.6 percent; relative risk, 0.77; P<0.001), and complications related to diabetes (6.4 percent vs. 7.6 percent; relative risk, 0.84; P=0.03).

CONCLUSIONS:

Ramipril significantly reduces the rates of death, myocardial infarction, and stroke in a broad range of high-risk patients who are not known to have a low ejection fraction or heart failure

ON TARGET TRIAL

TELMISARTAN, RAMIPRIL, OR BOTH IN PATIENTS AT HIGH RISK FOR VASCULAR EVENTS. NEW ENGLAND JOURNAL OF MEDICINE (NEJM) 2008.

This trial was trying to assess the role of angiotensin-receptor blockers (ARBs) in patients who were at high risk for cardiovascular events but who did not have left ventricular dysfunction or heart failure and whether there is any benefit from combining ARBs with ACEI in such patients. The trial compared the ACE inhibitor ramipril, the ARB telmisartan, and the combination of the two drugs in patients with vascular disease or high-risk diabetes. Results showed that Telmisartan was equivalent to ramipril in patients with vascular disease or high-risk diabetes and was associated with less angioedema. However, the combination of the two drugs was associated with more adverse events with no additional benefit.

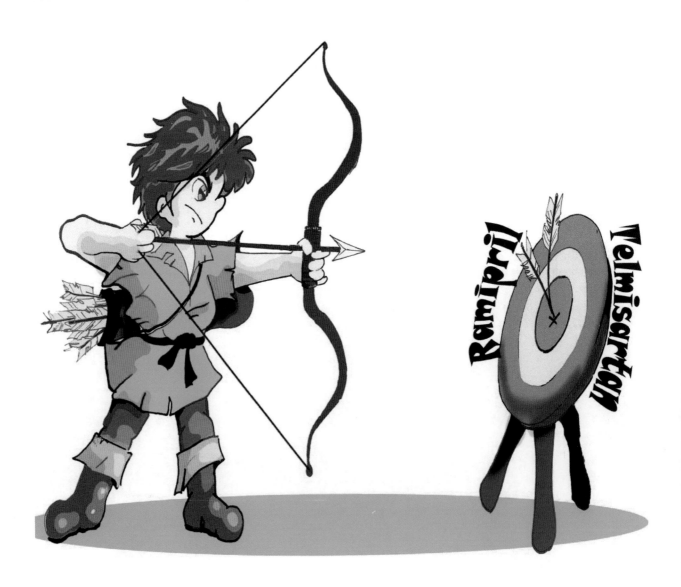

ONTARGET TRIAL

Telmisartan, ramipril, or both in patients at high risk for vascular events.

Yusuf S, et al. ONTARGET Investigators.

New England Journal of Medicine (NEJM) 2008; April 10; 358(15):1547-59.

BACKGROUND:

In patients who have vascular disease or high-risk diabetes without heart failure, angiotensin-converting-enzyme (ACE) inhibitors reduce mortality and morbidity from cardiovascular causes, but the role of angiotensin-receptor blockers (ARBs) in such patients is unknown. We compared the ACE inhibitor ramipril, the ARB telmisartan, and the combination of the two drugs in patients with vascular disease or high-risk diabetes.

METHODS:

After a 3-week, single-blind run-in period, patients underwent double-blind randomization, with 8576 assigned to receive 10 mg of ramipril per day, 8542 assigned to receive 80 mg of telmisartan per day, and 8502 assigned to receive both drugs (combination therapy). The primary composite outcome was death from cardiovascular causes, myocardial infarction, stroke, or hospitalization for heart failure.

RESULTS:

Mean blood pressure was lower in both the telmisartan group (a 0.9/0.6 mm Hg greater reduction) and the combination-therapy group (a 2.4/1.4 mm Hg greater reduction) than in the ramipril group. At a median follow-up of 56 months, the primary outcome had occurred in 1412 patients in the ramipril group (16.5%), as compared with 1423 patients in the telmisartan group (16.7%; relative risk, 1.01; 95% confidence interval [CI], 0.94 to 1.09). As compared with the ramipril group, the telmisartan group had lower rates of cough (1.1% vs. 4.2%, P<0.001) and angioedema (0.1% vs. 0.3%, P=0.01) and a higher rate of hypotensive symptoms (2.6% vs. 1.7%, P<0.001); the rate of syncope was the same in the two groups (0.2%). In the combination-therapy group, the primary outcome occurred in 1386 patients (16.3%; relative risk, 0.99; 95% CI, 0.92 to 1.07); as compared with the ramipril group, there was an increased risk of hypotensive symptoms (4.8% vs. 1.7%, P<0.001), syncope (0.3% vs. 0.2%, P=0.03), and renal dysfunction (13.5% vs. 10.2%, P<0.001).

CONCLUSIONS:

Telmisartan was equivalent to ramipril in patients with vascular disease or high-risk diabetes and was associated with less angioedema. The combination of the two drugs was associated with more adverse events without an increase in benefit.

CARISA AND MARISA TRIALS

Ranolazine is believed to inhibit fatty acid oxidation, shift metabolism toward carbohydrate oxidation, and increase the efficiency of oxygen use. These effects may lead to an increase exercise performance in patients with chronic angina. The safety and efficacy of the drug was tested initially in two trials CARISA and MARISA. CARISA trial was performed to determine whether, at trough levels will improve exercise tolerance in patients who still have chronic angina in spite of optimal medical therapy, and Ranolazine was shown to provide additional antianginal relief in this population. MARISA trial on the other hand tested the dose-response relationship of ranolazine and showed an increase in the exercise duration with the increased dose of ranolazine without hemodynamic compromise .

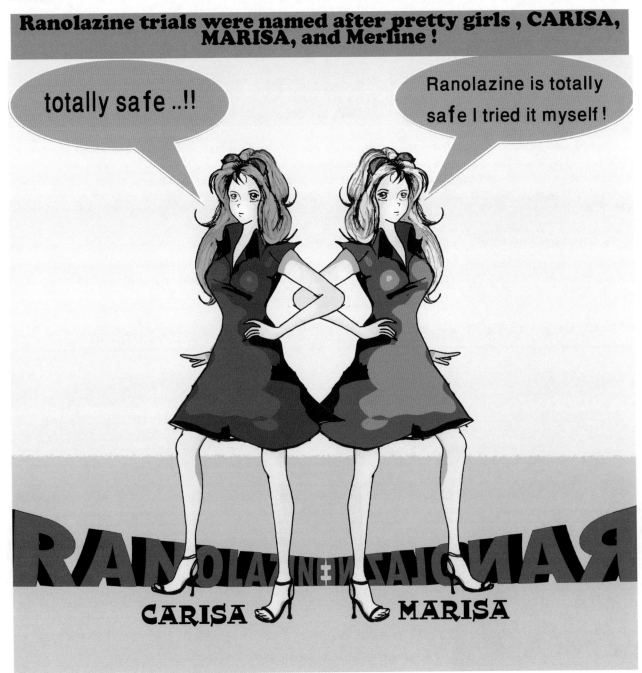

190

CARISA TRIAL
Effects of ranolazine with atenolol, amlodipine, or diltiazem on exercise tolerance and angina frequency in patients with severe chronic angina: a randomized controlled trial.
Chaitman BR, et al.
Combination Assessment of Ranolazine In Stable Angina (CARISA) Investigators.
Journal of the American Medical Association (JAMA). 2004; January 21;291(3):309-16.

CONTEXT: Many patients with chronic angina experience anginal episodes despite revascularization and antianginal medications. In a previous trial, antianginal monotherapy with ranolazine, a drug believed to partially inhibit fatty acid oxidation, increased treadmill exercise performance; however, its long-term efficacy and safety have not been studied in combination with beta-blockers or calcium antagonists in a large patient population with severe chronic angina.

OBJECTIVES: To determine whether, at trough levels, ranolazine improves the total exercise time of patients who have symptoms of chronic angina and who experience angina and ischemia at low workloads despite taking standard doses of atenolol, amlodipine, or diltiazem and to determine times to angina onset and to electrocardiographic evidence of myocardial ischemia, effect on angina attacks and nitroglycerin use, and effect on long-term survival in an open-label observational study extension.

DESIGN, SETTING, AND PATIENTS: A randomized, 3-group parallel, double-blind, placebo-controlled trial of 823 eligible adults with symptomatic chronic angina who were randomly assigned to receive placebo or 1 of 2 doses of ranolazine. Patients treated at the 118 participating ambulatory outpatient settings in several countries were enrolled in the Combination Assessment of Ranolazine In Stable Angina (CARISA) trial from July 1999 to August 2001 and followed up through October 31, 2002.

INTERVENTION: Patients received twice-daily placebo or 750 mg or 1000 mg of ranolazine. Treadmill exercise 12 hours (trough) and 4 hours (peak) after dosing was assessed after 2, 6 (t ough only), and 12 weeks of treatment.

MAIN OUTCOME MEASURES: Change in exercise duration, time to onset of angina, time to onset of ischemia, nitroglycerin use, and number of angina attacks.

RESULTS: Trough exercise duration increased by 115.6 seconds from baseline in both ranolazine groups (pooled) vs 91.7 seconds in the placebo group (P =.01). The times to angina and to electrocardiographic ischemia also increased in the ranolazine groups, at peak more than at trough. The increases did not depend on changes in blood pressure, heart rate, or background antianginal therapy and persisted throughout 12 weeks. Ranolazine reduced angina attacks and nitroglycerin use by about 1 per week vs placebo (P<.02). Survival of 750 patients taking ranolazine during the CARISA trial or its associated long-term open-label study was 98.4% in the first year and 95.9% in the second year.

CONCLUSION: Twice-daily doses of ranolazine increased exercise capacity and provided additional antianginal relief to symptomatic patients with severe chronic angina taking standard doses of atenolol, amlodipine, or diltiazem, without evident adverse, long-term survival consequences over 1 to 2 years of therapy.

MARISA Trial
Anti-ischemic effects and long-term survival during ranolazine monotherapy in patients with chronic severe angina.
Chaitman BR, et al MARISA Investigators.
Journal of the American College of Cardiology 2004; April 21;43(8):1375-82.

OBJECTIVES: The primary objective of the Monotherapy Assessment of Ranolazine In Stable Angina (MARISA) trial was to determine the dose-response relationship of ranolazine, a potentially new anti-anginal compound, on symptom-limited exercise duration.

BACKGROUND: Fatty acids rise precipitously in response to stress, including acute myocardial ischemia. Ranolazine is believed to partially inhibit fatty acid oxidation, shift metabolism toward carbohydrate oxidation, and increase the efficiency of oxygen use.

METHODS: Patients (n = 191) with angina-limited exercise discontinued anti-anginal medications and were randomized into a double-blind four-period crossover study of sustained-release ranolazine 500, 1,000, or 1,500 mg, or placebo, each administered twice daily for one week. Exercise testing was performed at the end of each treatment during both trough and peak ranolazine plasma concentrations.

RESULTS: Exercise duration at trough increased with ranolazine 500, 1,000, and 1,500 mg twice daily by 94, 103, and 116 s, respectively, all greater (p < 0.005) than the 70-s increase on placebo. Dose-related increases in exercise duration at peak and in times to 1 mm ST-segment depression at trough and peak and to angina at trough and peak were also demonstrated (all p < 0.005). Ranolazine had negligible effects on heart rate and blood pressure. One year survival rate combining data from the MARISA trial and its open-label follow-on study was 96.3 +/- 1.7%.

CONCLUSIONS: In chronic angina patients, ranolazine monotherapy was well tolerated and increased exercise performance throughout its dosing interval at all doses studied without clinically meaningful hemodynamic effects. One-year survival was not lower than expected in this high-risk patient population. This metabolic approach to treating myocardial ischemia may offer a new therapeutic option for chronic angina patients.

CHARISMA TRIAL

CLOPIDOGREL AND ASPIRIN VERSUS ASPIRIN ALONE FOR THE PREVENTION OF ATHEROTHROMBOTIC EVENTS.
NEW ENGLAND JOURNAL OF MEDICINE (NEJM) 2006.

CHARISMA trial hypothesized that dual anti-platelet therapy with clopidogrel plus aspirin might be beneficial as prophylactic measures in patients with multiple risk factors for cardiovascular disease. It was found that this treatment compared to aspirin alone, is not only not beneficial rather it might be harmful, increasing the risk of bleeding in patients who only carry risk factors and no evidence of symptomatic cardiovascular disease

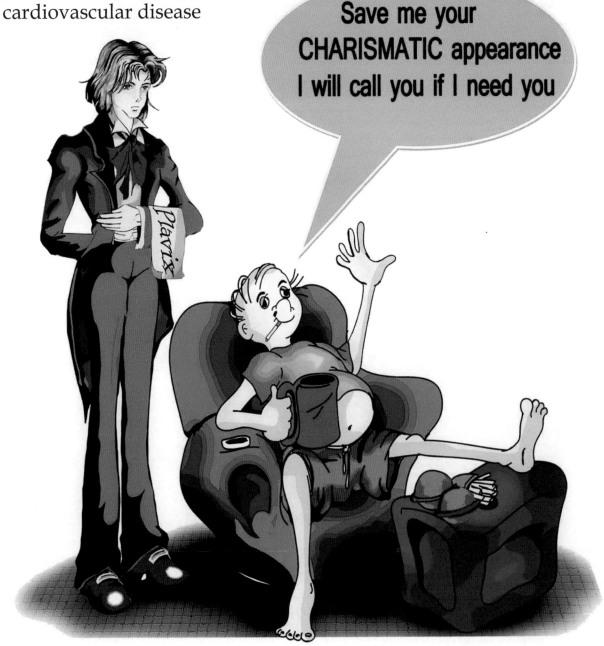

Save me your CHARISMATIC appearance I will call you if I need you

CHARISMA TRIAL

Clopidogrel and aspirin versus aspirin alone for the prevention of atherothrombotic events. Bhatt DL, el al.

New England Journal of Medicine (NEJM) 2006; April 20; 354(16):1706-17.

BACKGROUND:

Dual antiplatelet therapy with clopidogrel plus low-dose aspirin has not been studied in a broad population of patients at high risk for atherothrombotic events.

METHODS:

We randomly assigned 15,603 patients with either clinically evident cardiovascular disease or multiple risk factors to receive clopidogrel (75 mg per day) plus low-dose aspirin (75 to 162 mg per day) or placebo plus low-dose aspirin and followed them for a median of 28 months. The primary efficacy end point was a composite of myocardial infarction, stroke, or death from cardiovascular causes.

RESULTS:

The rate of the primary efficacy end point was 6.8 percent with clopidogrel plus aspirin and 7.3 percent with placebo plus aspirin (relative risk, 0.93; 95 percent confidence interval, 0.83 to 1.05; P=0.22). The respective rate of the principal secondary efficacy end point, which included hospitalizations for ischemic events, was 16.7 percent and 17.9 percent (relative risk, 0.92; 95 percent confidence interval, 0.86 to 0.995; P=0.04), and the rate of severe bleeding was 1.7 percent and 1.3 percent (relative risk, 1.25; 95 percent confidence interval, 0.97 to 1.61 percent; P=0.09). The rate of the primary end point among patients with multiple risk factors was 6.6 percent with clopidogrel and 5.5 percent with placebo (relative risk, 1.2; 95 percent confidence interval, 0.91 to 1.59; P=0.20) and the rate of death from cardiovascular causes also was higher with clopidogrel (3.9 percent vs. 2.2 percent, P=0.01). In the subgroup with clinically evident atherothrombosis, the rate was 6.9 percent with clopidogrel and 7.9 percent with placebo (relative risk, 0.88; 95 percent confidence interval, 0.77 to 0.998; P=0.046).

CONCLUSIONS:

In this trial, there was a suggestion of benefit with clopidogrel treatment in patients with symptomatic atherothrombosis and a suggestion of harm in patients with multiple risk factors. Overall, clopidogrel plus aspirin was not significantly more effective than aspirin alone in reducing the rate of myocardial infarction, stroke, or death from cardiovascular causes.

COURAGE TRIAL

OPTIMAL MEDICAL THERAPY WITH OR WITHOUT PCI FOR STABLE CORONARY DISEASE.
NEW ENGLAND JOURNAL OF MEDICINE (NEJM) 2007.

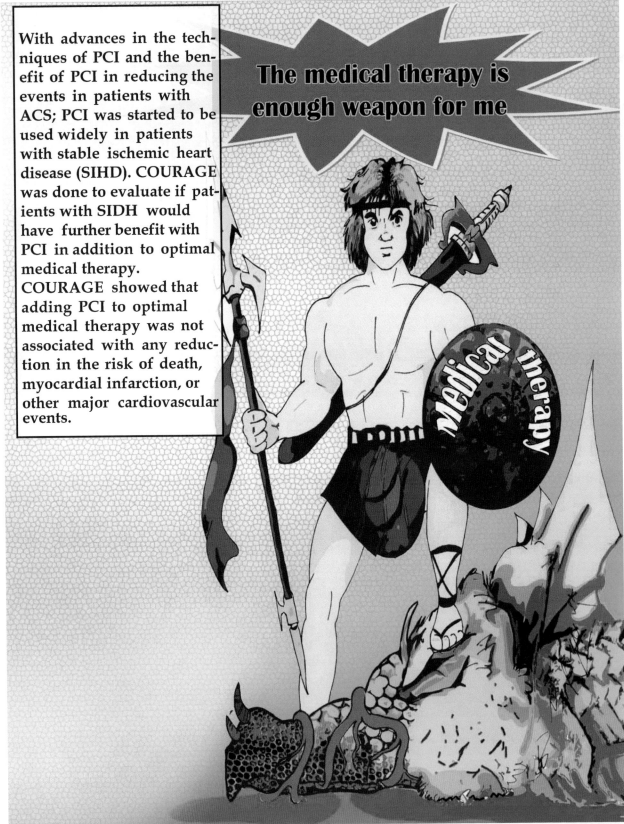

With advances in the techniques of PCI and the benefit of PCI in reducing the events in patients with ACS; PCI was started to be used widely in patients with stable ischemic heart disease (SIHD). COURAGE was done to evaluate if patients with SIDH would have further benefit with PCI in addition to optimal medical therapy.

COURAGE showed that adding PCI to optimal medical therapy was not associated with any reduction in the risk of death, myocardial infarction, or other major cardiovascular events.

The medical therapy is enough weapon for me

Medical therapy

COURAGE TRIAL
Optimal medical therapy with or without PCI for stable coronary disease.
Boden WE, et al.

New England Journal of Medicine (NEJM) 2007; April 12; 356(15):1503-16..

BACKGROUND:

In patients with stable coronary artery disease, it remains unclear whether an initial management strategy of percutaneous coronary intervention (PCI) with intensive pharmacologic therapy and lifestyle intervention (optimal medical therapy) is superior to optimal medical therapy alone in reducing the risk of cardiovascular events.

METHODS:

We conducted a randomized trial involving 2287 patients who had objective evidence of myocardial ischemia and significant coronary artery disease at 50 U.S. and Canadian centers. Between 1999 and 2004, we assigned 1149 patients to undergo PCI with optimal medical therapy (PCI group) and 1138 to receive optimal medical therapy alone (medical-therapy group). The primary outcome was death from any cause and nonfatal myocardial infarction during a follow-up period of 2.5 to 7.0 years (median, 4.6).

RESULTS:

There were 211 primary events in the PCI group and 202 events in the medical-therapy group. The 4.6-year cumulative primary-event rates were 19.0% in the PCI group and 18.5% in the medical-therapy group (hazard ratio for the PCI group, 1.05; 95% confidence interval [CI], 0.87 to 1.27; P=0.62). There were no significant differences between the PCI group and the medical-therapy group in the composite of death, myocardial infarction, and stroke (20.0% vs. 19.5%; hazard ratio, 1.05; 95% CI, 0.87 to 1.27; P=0.62); hospitalization for acute coronary syndrome (12.4% vs. 11.8%; hazard ratio, 1.07; 95% CI, 0.84 to 1.37; P=0.56); or myocardial infarction (13.2% vs. 12.3%; hazard ratio, 1.13; 95% CI, 0.89 to 1.43; P=0.33).

CONCLUSIONS:

As an initial management strategy in patients with stable coronary artery disease, PCI did not reduce the risk of death, myocardial infarction, or other major cardiovascular events when added to optimal medical therapy.

BARI TRIAL
THE FINAL 10-YEAR FOLLOW-UP RESULTS FROM THE BARI RANDOMIZED TRIAL.
BARI INVESTIGATORS.
JOURNAL OF THE AMERICAN COLLEGE OF CARDIOLOGY. 2007.

This study was done to compare angioplasty and bypass surgery in symptomatic patients with multivessel coronary artery disease. After almost 10 years of follow-up there was no significant long-term disadvantage regarding mortality or myocardial infarction associated with an initial strategy of PTCA compared with CABG. Except among diabetic patients where CABG offered long-term survival benefit.

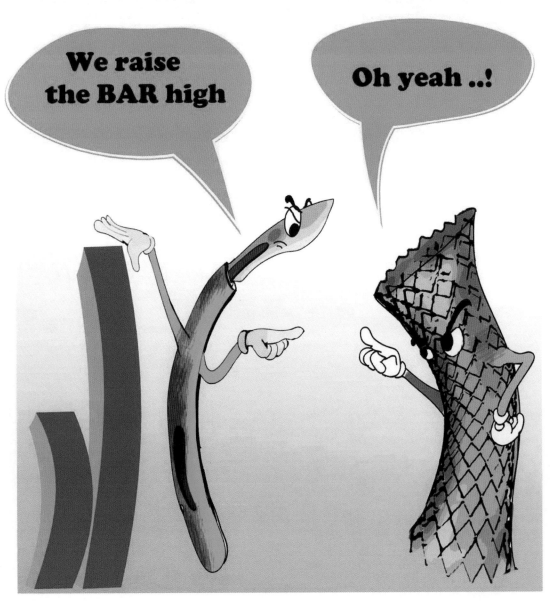

BARI Trial
The final 10-year follow-up results from the BARI randomized trial.
BARI Investigators.

Journal of the American College of Cardiology. 2007; April 17; 49(15):1600-6.

OBJECTIVES

We sought to compare 10-year clinical outcomes in the BARI (Bypass Angioplasty Revascularization Investigation) trial patients who were randomly assigned to percutaneous transluminal coronary balloon angioplasty (PTCA) versus coronary artery bypass grafting (CABG).

BACKGROUND

Angioplasty and bypass surgery have been compared in numerous studies, but long-term clinical outcomes are limited.

METHODS

Symptomatic patients with multivessel coronary artery disease (n = 1,829) were randomly assigned to initial treatment with PTCA or CABG and followed up for an average of 10.4 years. Analyses were conducted on an intention-to-treat basis.

RESULTS

The 10-year survival was 71.0% for PTCA and 73.5% for CABG (p = 0.18). At 10 years, the PTCA group had substantially higher subsequent revascularization rates than the CABG group (76.8% vs. 20.3%, p < 0.001), but angina rates for the 2 groups were similar. In the subgroup of patients with no treated diabetes, survival rates were nearly identical by randomization (PTCA 77.0% vs. CABG 77.3%, p = 0.59). In the subgroup with treated diabetes, the CABG assigned group had higher survival than the PTCA assigned group (PTCA 45.5% vs. CABG 57.8%, p = 0.025).

CONCLUSIONS

There was no significant long-term disadvantage regarding mortality or myocardial infarction associated with an initial strategy of PTCA compared with CABG. Among patients with treated diabetes, CABG conferred long-term survival benefit, whereas the 2 initial strategies were equivalent regarding survival for patients without diabetes.

SYNTAX TRIAL

PERCUTANEOUS CORONARY INTERVENTION VERSUS CORONARY-ARTERY BYPASS GRAFTING FOR SEVERE CORONARY ARTERY DISEASE.
NEW ENGLAND JOURNAL OF MEDICINE (NEJM). 2009.

The first randomized clinical trial performed to compare outcomes of revascularization with PCI with drug-eluding stents (DES) vs. CABG in patients with multivessel coronary artery disease. SYNTAX showed that patients undergoing PCI were more likely to have repeat revascularization, while the rates of death and myocardial infarction were similar between the two groups; stroke was significantly more likely to occur with CABG. for patients with three-vessel or left main coronary disease, CABG remains the standard of care.

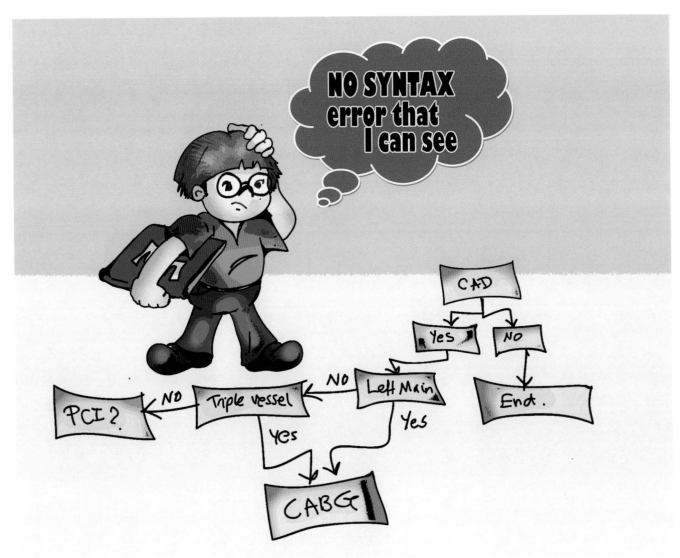

SYNTAX TRIAL

Percutaneous coronary intervention versus coronary-artery bypass grafting for severe coronary artery disease.

Serruys PW, et al. SYNTAX Investigators.

New England Journal of Medicine (NEJM). 2009; March 5; 360(10):961-72.

BACKGROUND:

Percutaneous coronary intervention (PCI) involving drug-eluting stents is increasingly used to treat complex coronary artery disease, although coronary-artery bypass grafting (CABG) has been the treatment of choice historically. Our trial compared PCI and CABG for treating patients with previously untreated three-vessel or left main coronary artery disease (or both).

METHODS:

We randomly assigned 1800 patients with three-vessel or left main coronary artery disease to undergo CABG or PCI (in a 1:1 ratio). For all these patients, the local cardiac surgeon and interventional cardiologist determined that equivalent anatomical revascularization could be achieved with either treatment. A noninferiority comparison of the two groups was performed for the primary end point--a major adverse cardiac or cerebrovascular event (i.e., death from any cause, stroke, myocardial infarction, or repeat revascularization) during the 12-month period after randomization. Patients for whom only one of the two treatment options would be beneficial, because of anatomical features or clinical conditions, were entered into a parallel, nested CABG or PCI registry.

RESULTS:

Most of the preoperative characteristics were similar in the two groups. Rates of major adverse cardiac or cerebrovascular events at 12 months were significantly higher in the PCI group (17.8%, vs. 12.4% for CABG; P=0.002), in large part because of an increased rate of repeat revascularization (13.5% vs. 5.9%, P<0.001); as a result, the criterion for noninferiority was not met. At 12 months, the rates of death and myocardial infarction were similar between the two groups; stroke was significantly more likely to occur with CABG (2.2%, vs. 0.6% with PCI; P=0.003).

CONCLUSIONS:

CABG remains the standard of care for patients with three-vessel or left main coronary artery disease, since the use of CABG, as compared with PCI, resulted in lower rates of the combined end point of major adverse cardiac or cerebrovascular events at 1 year.

FREEDOM TRIAL
FARKOUH ME, ET AL. STRATEGIES FOR MULTIVESSEL REVASCULARIZATION IN PATIENTS WITH DIABETES.
NEW ENGLAND JOURNAL OF MEDICINE (NEJM) 2012.

SYNTAX showed that CABG was the preferred strategy for patients with three-vessel or left main coronary artery disease. Subsequently a subgroup analysis showed the benefit that CABG offer in patients with multi-vessel disease was more prominent in diabetic patients. FREEDOM was done to compare outcomes of revascularization with PCI with DES vs. CABG specifically in diabetic patient with multivessel coronary artery disease. FREEDOM confirmed that CABG should remain the standard of care for patients with three-vessel and diabetes as it significantly reduced rates of death and myocardial infarction when compared with PCI.

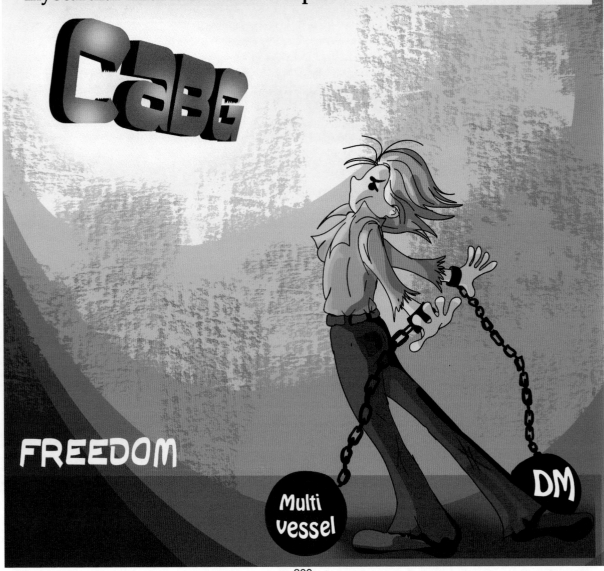

FREEDOM TRIAL

Strategies for multivessel revascularization in patients with diabetes.
Farkouh ME, et al.

New England Journal of Medicine (NEJM) 2012; December 20; 367(25):2375-84.

BACKGROUND:

In some randomized trials comparing revascularization strategies for patients with diabetes, coronary-artery bypass grafting (CABG) has had a better outcome than percutaneous coronary intervention (PCI). We sought to discover whether aggressive medical therapy and the use of drug-eluting stents could alter the revascularization approach for patients with diabetes and multivessel coronary artery disease.

METHODS:

In this randomized trial, we assigned patients with diabetes and multivessel coronary artery disease to undergo either PCI with drug-eluting stents or CABG. The patients were followed for a minimum of 2 years (median among survivors, 3.8 years). All patients were prescribed currently recommended medical therapies for the control of low-density lipoprotein cholesterol, systolic blood pressure, and glycated hemoglobin. The primary outcome measure was a composite of death from any cause, nonfatal myocardial infarction, or nonfatal stroke.

RESULTS:

From 2005 through 2010, we enrolled 1900 patients at 140 international centers. The patients' mean age was 63.1±9.1 years, 29% were women, and 83% had three-vessel disease. The primary outcome occurred more frequently in the PCI group (P=0.005), with 5-year rates of 26.6% in the PCI group and 18.7% in the CABG group. The benefit of CABG was driven by differences in rates of both myocardial infarction (P<0.001) and death from any cause (P=0.049). Stroke was more frequent in the CABG group, with 5-year rates of 2.4% in the PCI group and 5.2% in the CABG group (P=0.03).

CONCLUSIONS:

For patients with diabetes and advanced coronary artery disease, CABG was superior to PCI in that it significantly reduced rates of death and myocardial infarction, with a higher rate of stroke.

PARTNER TRIAL

TRANSCATHETER AORTIC-VALVE IMPLANTATION FOR AORTIC STENOSIS IN PATIENTS WHO CANNOT UNDERGO SURGERY.
NEW ENGLAND JOURNAL OF MEDICINE (NEJM) 2010.

Transcatheter aortic-valve implantation (TAVI) was introduced as an alternative to surgical replacement in patients with sever aortic stenosis, who are not suitable for surgical intervention. PARTNER trial demonstrated that TAVI, as compared with standard therapy, significantly reduced the rates of death from any cause, or repeat hospitalization, and cardiac symptoms, despite the higher incidence of major strokes and major vascular complications .

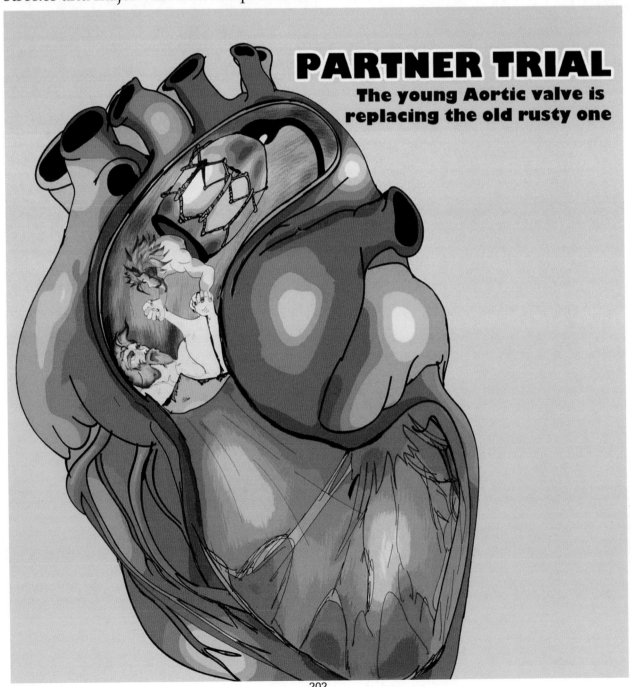

PARTNER TRIAL
The young Aortic valve is replacing the old rusty one

PARTNER TRIAL

Transcatheter aortic-valve implantation for aortic stenosis in patients who cannot undergo surgery.

Leon MB, et al. PARTNER Trial Investigators.

New England Journal of Medicine (NEJM) 2010; October 21; 363(17):1597-607.

BACKGROUND:

Many patients with severe aortic stenosis and coexisting conditions are not candidates for surgical replacement of the aortic valve. Recently, transcatheter aortic-valve implantation (TAVI) has been suggested as a less invasive treatment for high-risk patients with aortic stenosis.

METHODS:

We randomly assigned patients with severe aortic stenosis, whom surgeons considered not to be suitable candidates for surgery, to standard therapy (including balloon aortic valvuloplasty) or transfemoral transcatheter implantation of a balloon-expandable bovine pericardial valve. The primary end point was the rate of death from any cause.

RESULTS:

A total of 358 patients with aortic stenosis who were not considered to be suitable candidates for surgery underwent randomization at 21 centers (17 in the United States). At 1 year, the rate of death from any cause (Kaplan–Meier analysis) was 30.7% with TAVI, as compared with 50.7% with standard therapy (hazard ratio with TAVI, 0.55; 95% confidence interval [CI], 0.40 to 0.74; P<0.001). The rate of the composite end point of death from any cause or repeat hospitalization was 42.5% with TAVI as compared with 71.6% with standard therapy (hazard ratio, 0.46; 95% CI, 0.35 to 0.59; P<0.001). Among survivors at 1 year, the rate of cardiac symptoms (New York Heart Association class III or IV) was lower among patients who had undergone TAVI than among those who had received standard therapy (25.2% vs. 58.0%, P<0.001). At 30 days, TAVI, as compared with standard therapy, was associated with a higher incidence of major strokes (5.0% vs. 1.1%, P=0.06) and major vascular complications (16.2% vs. 1.1%, P<0.001). In the year after TAVI, there was no deterioration in the functioning of the bioprosthetic valve, as assessed by evidence of stenosis or regurgitation on an echocardiogram.

CONCLUSIONS:

In patients with severe aortic stenosis who were not suitable candidates for surgery, TAVI, as compared with standard therapy, significantly reduced the rates of death from any cause, the composite end point of death from any cause or repeat hospitalization, and cardiac symptoms, despite the higher incidence of major strokes and major vascular events.

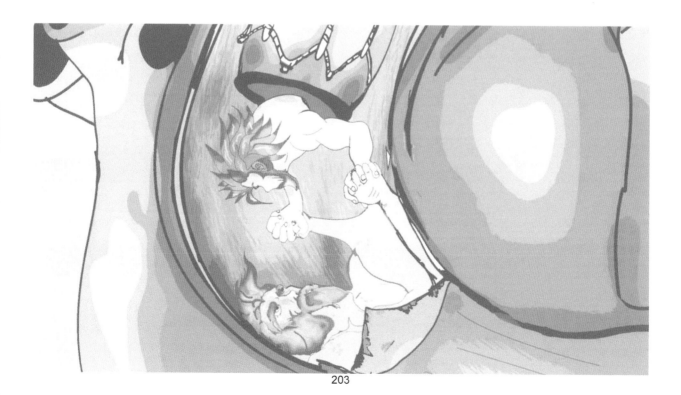

Made in the USA
Lexington, KY
26 May 2015